MW00953215

Table of Contents

Chapter 1: The improved cabbage soup diet 2.0 revealed 5

Why Soup Diets work!...9

The Concentrated Power of Cabbage Nutrition..............................9

Chapter 2: Prepare yourself for success before starting the Cabbage Soup Diet 11

5 important aspects about keeping your metabolism running.......11

Ten golden rules for better results..16

The best day to start with your cabbage soup diet........................19

Safe foods that let you "cheat" and not have to worry about 21

The 3 biggest traps, you should be prepared for as dieter 22

Chapter 3: Reduce any side effects during the Cabbage Soup Diet 2.0 - Or avoid them all together! 24

The evolution of the Cabbage Soup Diet 2.0...................................24

The ultimate protein shake - a metabolism booster.......................26

Safety on the Cabbage Soup Diet...28

Getting past the Day 2 hump 29

Coffee and Dieting 30

The Cabbage Soup Diet 2.0 plan overview....................................32

Day 1 - Fruit Day...34

Day 2 - Vegetable Day 37

Day 3 - Fruit and Vegetable Day..40

Day 4 - Banana Day 42

Day 5 - Fish & Tomato Day 44

Day 6 - Meat Day...47

Day 7 - Rice Day..49

Master your cravings in just days - and never rely on willpower alone to lose weight again! 52

Keeping up motivation during the diet week..............................55

Keep a diet journal 55

8 ways to get rid of fattening toxins 59

Lower your toxic load..59

The top 7 most common mistakes...66

How to reduce common side effects like headache and fatigue 72

10 bonus tips for best results...73

Frequent questions from my readers 74

Chapter 4: Cook delicious cabbage soup the fast and easy way! 77

Delicious Cabbage Soup Recipe Variations 79

Reduce flatulence, aches and pains 81

Save 80% of your preparation and cooking time - and save money! 82

Freezing Your Cabbage Soup..84

Frequent questions from my readers 85

Chapter 5: How to avoid bad old habits after the Cabbage Soup Diet 87

The No.1 maintenance tip after the cabbage soup diet 2.0............87

The Dramatic Satiety Difference between Soup and Water 88

The most important ingredient after the cabbage soup diet..........90

The single biggest mistake after finishing the Cabbage Soup Diet .92

My Top 5 motivation techniques for enhancing & maintaining a "thin you" 93

Simple, healthy ways to improve your diet.........................95

Chapter 6: The essentials of keeping the new you - long after you've finished the Cabbage Soup Diet 2.0!...............................99

Diet traps to avoid in every situation 99

Some goldmines for fast food junkies.............................102

Healthy Breakfast Ideas 103

Sweet facts - What you must know about sugar and carbohydrates
....105

Understanding Glycemic Load vs. Glycemic Index 110

All About Artificial Sweeteners 113

Healthy ways to satisfy your sweet tooth 114

Get The Real Facts About Food & Detect Food Manipulation 115

Developing a lasting weight loss concept 118

Stay on track today, tomorrow, and for the rest of your life 125

Following the Healthy Eating Pyramid guidelines 129

The Building Blocks of the Healthy Eating Pyramid.......................129

15 more tips to KEEP the NEW YOU permanently! 131

Some final words 135

One last thought 136

<u>IMPORTANT SAFETY INFORMATION</u>

AS WITH ANY OTHER DIET, YOU SHOULD CONSULT YOUR DOCTOR BEFORE BEGINNING THE CABBAGE SOUP DIET. THIS IS PARTICULARLY IMPORTANT IF YOU ARE SUFFERING FROM AN ILLNESS OR TAKING MEDICATION. FURTHERMORE, YOU SHOULD ONLY REMAIN ON THIS WEIGHT LOSS PROGRAM FOR ONE WEEK AT A TIME AS THE CABBAGE SOUP DIET 2.0 IS NOT APPROPRIATE FOR LONG-TERM USE.

SWITCH TO HEALTHY, LONG-TERM NUTRITION AFTER THE DIET WEEK AND ALLOW AT LEAST THREE MONTHS BEFORE RETURNING TO THE CABBAGE SOUP DIET 2.0. IF YOU WANT TO REPEAT THE DIET DON'T DO SO MORE THAN 3 - 4 TIMES PER YEAR; ALWAYS WITH 3 MONTH INTERVALS BETWEEN DIETING.

UNDER NO CIRCUMSTANCES IS THIS DIET APPROPRIATE FOR CHILDREN OR ADOLESCENTS.

The Cabbage Soup Diet 2.0 – a perfect decision

A heartfelt welcome to you and congratulations on taking this brave step towards successful dieting that will save you much pain, money and time. You have just chosen the one book that can change your life forever! If you're ready to reach for your dream of weight loss, then the Cabbage Soup Diet 2.0 will help you switch on to a healthy lifestyle you never dreamed you could achieve.

In my step-by-step guide I'll show you exactly how to prepare yourself <u>before</u> starting the Cabbage Soup Diet. I've covered what to do <u>during</u> and <u>right after</u> the diet week and how to keep the new you <u>long after</u> you've finished this jump-start diet concept.

Health fads come and go, but for more than three decades the Cabbage Soup Diet has been a slimming sensation. For every jealous doctor and weight loss expert who has tried to keep their patients or customers in the dark about this diet, there are more than 1000 Cabbage Soup Dieters who are living proof that **the Cabbage Soup Diet <u>really</u> works**. There are several versions of the cabbage soup diet that have come to light in the last decades under different names, with a new version now: **The Cabbage Soup Diet 2.0.** So why a new version?

The Cabbage Soup Diet 2.0 represents both an old and a very new approach to weight loss with cabbage soup.

It is old in that I have built upon a successful approach to slimming of unknown origin, developed in the late 70's. The old style cabbage soup diet has been an enduring slimming sensation for more than 30 years.

The Cabbage Soup Diet 2.0 is new in that I've applied cutting edge research to the enduring cabbage soup diet plan. I've included the phenomenal feedback I received from my website readers over the years, optimizing the diet to the greatest degree possible. Last, but definitely not least, I've added scientific research and proof of how the diet works wherever possible.

Lose up to 10 pounds per week with no muscle loss!

The Cabbage Soup Diet 2.0 will allow dieters to lose up to 10 pounds per week with no muscle loss. With this improved version it's now easier than ever to jump start your weight loss efforts and get the motivation you need to succeed long-term. What's more, the cabbage soup diet 2.0 is hunger-proof! You can lose weight while still having plenty of filling, delicious, and nutritious foods.

Here are the benefits offered by this Cabbage Soup Diet 2.0 manual:

- Discover how to get the best results from the Cabbage Soup Diet by following the 3 day preparation guide for **before** you start

- Find out about the 5 most important keys to keeping your metabolism running on high & burning fat for lasting weight loss results.

- Get my personal tips on how to master cravings and control the urge to overeat

- Understand the 3 biggest dieting traps & 7 most common dieting mistakes - so you can avoid these traps and truly achieve success

- I'll reveal my 10 golden rules for better results - PLUS my 10 bonus tips - so nothing in your diet is left to chance!

- Find out how you can get past the 2 day hump to stay on track to your weight loss goal

- Discover some 'cheats' that you can eat while doing the Cabbage Soup Diet - so you can curb any cravings without impacting on the cleansing process or your results!

- I'll show you how to adapt the Cabbage Soup Diet plan if you're vegetarian & give away some delicious vegetarian recipes to use while dieting

- Uncover the single most essential element on the Cabbage Soup Diet - with this vital 'ingredient' you can dramatically boost your diet results!

I've worked on pulling out even the smallest secrets and hints that I've learned over the years and I'll tell you precisely which tools you need to jumpstart your weight loss - and keep the pounds of for good.

Make a strong start

We so often hear the term "slow and steady wins the race", believing that with this approach we will have more success. However, there is now evidence to show a slow-working diet of any kind is among the **least** effective weight-loss plans. When a slow diet turns you off at the beginning, when you are most eager to see signs of success, then it is at this time that many dieters fail. When you are dieting, it is at the beginning when quick weight loss and motivation matter most.

In recent studies it has been shown that dieters who lost weight quickly and lost more total weight were the ones who kept off more weight in the long-term. Researchers concluded that the first 2-4 weeks of the diet and the success in this time can predict dieters' future successes for up to five years.

My Cabbage Soup Diet 2.0 is a step-by-step guide, giving you precise guidelines and many hints so that nothing is left to chance.
If you follow the diet plan then there is no room for mistakes - it's that simple. In fact, following the rules in this book provides a virtual blueprint for success.

You can lose up to ten pounds in seven days and never feel hungry

While we can't predict the future, there is no doubt that by following this diet and experiencing impressive weight loss during the first seven days, you'll have a higher chance of breaking the diet/binge cycle forever. Once you master this, you'll be on track to live a healthier, more satisfying life.

Why Soup Diets work!

Soup Diets can help you to rapidly shed those unwanted pounds. Once upon a time, soup was primarily prescribed to stimulate the appetite, not to suppress it - but not anymore! Today soup is one of the most reliable ways to shed unwanted pounds. How does it work? Well there are a bunch of reasons - but this culminates in shrinking burgeoning waistlines.

New research has shown that eating broth-based soup does reduce cravings for other foods. Added to that, soup is a great convenience food - so no more need to resort to snacking. Soup can be thick or thin, smooth or chunky. Your soup can be filled with the healthiest ingredients and power foods can be combined with soup effortlessly. When you use power foods such as cabbage, it will slow down carbohydrate absorption and help to prevent surges in the hormones which stimulate appetite.

The cabbage soup is useful, as soup 'tricks' the body. When you eat the soup, your body believes that you have consumed a larger number of calories than you have actually taken in. On top of that, the warmth and liquid of the soup fills you up quickly, preventing the desire to overeat.

To support this process, my recipes make extensive use of ingredients rich in soluble fiber, a key ingredient in reducing cravings and over active appetites.

With these soups, you'll be able to consume a minimal amount of calories, while still slowing down the body's carbohydrate absorption. This will help in keeping your appetite firmly under your control.

The Concentrated Power of Cabbage Nutrition

Now I want to be clear about this diet right from the beginning. The 7 day diet week outlined can also work when based on a vegetable soup. You can succeed WITHOUT cabbage too, but by using cabbage you can maximize the health benefits achieved, as well as the amount of weight lost. Why?

Cabbage is rich in a wide range of vitamins and other nutrients that are healthy for your body. This vegetable is also a good source of vitamin A, all of the B vitamins, vitamins C and E, as well as calcium, selenium, potassium, magnesium and iron.

If the nutritional value is not enough, cabbage contains a wealth of dietary fiber as mentioned before, including the insoluble fiber cellulose. Humans cannot digest fiber, which means that fiber rich foods are great for increasing the bulk of stools and encouraging elimination of unwanted waste from the body.

In addition, cabbage is a vegetable that has a very low calorie content - just 15 calories in one cup. This power food has some protein and only a few carbohydrates, which means it doesn't encourage excess secretion of insulin - known as the "fat" hormone. The combination of all these attributes spells weight loss - making the Cabbage Soup Diet a winner and a must for dieters.

Cabbage is a food source that speeds up your metabolism naturally. This can help if dieters are also looking to eliminate drugs such as acetaminophen from their system. The release of such drugs at a faster rate can be beneficial as it ensures chemicals don't remain in the body longer than necessary. Cabbage has high iron and sulfur content as well, so it helps to cleanse your stomach and keep your gastrointestinal tract healthy. Furthermore, this magic vegetable encourages the clearing of mucous membranes in the intestine and eliminates fatty deposits as part of its fat burning effect.

Did I mention that cabbage is an inexpensive vegetable as well? If you don't want to blow the budget while losing weight, then the good news is that cabbage is relatively cheap - even though this vegetable is one of the richest sources of protective vitamins, minerals, phytochemicals and antioxidants –
all musts for good health. Adding cabbage to your diet and even a regular vegetable soup is ideal not only when you are aiming for weight loss.

Another major advantage of cabbage is that it offers a strong flavor that makes it ideal in a range of dishes.

Don't be afraid that eating cabbage will mean spooning up a tasteless, pale soup. I'll show you in chapter 4 how you can make it into a culinary delight.

Soup Diets & Cabbage – A magic combination

Your body needs a lot of energy to digest the cabbage soup - so you may wonder where does this energy come from? The simple answer is that your fat supplies it! On the Cabbage Soup Diet, there are foods that you're allowed to eat in unlimited quantities - and these are foods that will help your body to burn the maximum fat. You can avoid that 'empty feeling' by having plenty of the fruits and vegetables which actually provide fewer calories than your body uses in chewing, swallowing and digesting them!

It is this 'negative calorie load' that helps also explain why Cabbage Soup dieters can fill up on the soup 4 – 5 times a day - and still experience dramatic weight loss in just few days.

When you are on the Cabbage Soup Diet, your body is forced to work harder during digestion. This diet turns your body into a fat burning machine! No more starving... No more counting calories... Nothing but easy to follow weight loss!

Are you ready to jumpstart your weight loss?
Enjoy, good luck and watch the weight drop off!

Chapter 2: Prepare yourself for success before starting the Cabbage Soup Diet

5 important aspects about keeping your metabolism running

When you are aiming for the best possible results from your weight loss program, there are some important steps you need to follow to achieve the best results. If you get these wrong you could actually cause your metabolism to slow to a crawl. In order to avoid that from happening - here are some simple steps you can take to keep your metabolism running high and burning fat. Skipping or ignoring even one of these factors could mean your weight loss project is doomed to failure!

1) Eat sufficient amounts of the cabbage soup
2) Drink protein shakes during the course of the diet
3) Get moving - your body will look and feel better if you complement your diet with exercise
4) Maintain an effective Acid-Base balance - the right pH will help keep the weight loss going strong
5) Opt for low glycemic load foods

In order to help you understand the importance of each of these steps, I'd like to explain each one further.

1) Eat sufficient Cabbage Soup

As soon as you start the diet, make sure you don't start avoiding the cabbage soup too early in the process. There are some dieters who will avoid the soup as often as they can. This is completely the wrong approach and will stop you from reaching your goals. In other circumstances, people will have 1-2 portions of cabbage soup per day and they will feel this is enough.

Wrong! If you haven't fallen into the traps above, it doesn't finish there. Don't make the mistake of thinking you can consume the clear soup without the chunky parts. Wrong again! In order to get the best results you should consume one big pot of cabbage soup within two days. The 3-4 portions of cabbage soup per day is essential to your success. If you really don't like chunky soups, then think about mixing the soup in a blender so that you can eat the necessary amounts.

2) Drink protein shakes

While protein in present in cabbage, there is not enough available in the diet from the prototype cabbage soup diet plan alone. Protein is the substance our muscles are made from, it gives power and has fat melting properties.

Protein gives our body resources to exploit fat – and burn away fat deposits.

My Cabbage Soup Diet 2.0 plan takes the need for protein into account and allows 2 protein shakes per day. I can't stress enough that you must follow this step. If you don't give your body protein to burn fat it could end up melting your own muscle mass.

Either a soy or a whey protein shake will be suitable depending on your preference. To get the best results, opt for my ultimate protein shake recommendation, which boosts your energy and preserves muscle mass. You can find out more about this in chapter 3.

3) Move your body

Dieting alone is often not enough to achieve your weight loss goals effectively, so exercise is vital to your dieting success! Undertaking an exercise program is the ideal way to stimulate your metabolism. There are many different ways you can get moving and a broad range of physical activities that you can enjoy, many of which can be easily done without being expensive.

I suggest developing an exercise routine that fits into your daily schedule, so that you can manage it as an ongoing part of a healthy lifestyle. Determine the time of day in which you are most comfortable working-out and routinely set aside time for exercise. The ultimate time for your exercising is in the morning when your stomach is still empty. (Fasting and then exercising can really boost your results!)

If you're not used to routine exercise or you can't exercise for any reason, that's no problem! Your exercise routine needn't be an extensive workout - even a short, brisk walk once a day will help your overall health and increase your rate of weight loss. If you haven't exercised regularly in the past, then start off slowly and increase at your own pace. Don't forget that even small changes like parking farther from the door at the mall and taking stairs instead of the elevator can all add up when it comes to calorie-burning!

4) Acid-Base Balance

Under stress, not exercising, getting the wrong nutrition? If this sounds like where you're at right now, then your body is most likely producing acids. When you start dieting and increase the release of fat deposits, even more acid is produced, which can impair the body. With too much acid you could reduce your metabolism and decrease the catabolism of fat.

The consequences of this will be that your weight doesn't reduce or reduces very slowly. If you've done the cabbage soup diet and skipped this important check in the past, then this could mean you've lost considerably less weight than you had hoped for.

Test Your Body's Acidity or Alkalinity with pH Strips:

While you are doing the Cabbage Soup Diet, it is recommended that you test your body's pH levels to determine if whether or not this needs immediate attention. Using pH test strips, you can determine your pH factor quickly and easily in the privacy of your own home. A pH **below** 7.0 is acidic. A pH above 7.0 is alkaline. If your urinary pH fluctuates from 6.0 to 6.5 in the morning, and from 6.5 to 7.0 in the evening, then your body is functioning within a healthy range.

If the average urine pH is below 6.5, then the body's buffering system is overwhelmed and a state of "autotoxication" exists.

When this happens, you need to pay careful attention to the lower acid levels and start taking measures to correct this. Excess acids can be neutralized by the intake of vital, base substances which contain minerals and trace elements to excrete excess acids.

There are several products on the market that have a combination of base minerals and valuable trace elements. These components neutralize excess of acid and provide more energy and power. One example is AlkaMax pH Balance, but there are a number of others. If you're unsure, ask your local pharmacist.

5) Opt for low Glycemic Load Food

There are many popular diet books that include lists of foods based on the Glycemic Index (GI), and recommend avoiding all foods that have a high Glycemic Index.

Although the cabbage soup itself has a low Glycemic Index, some fruits like pineapples and melons are high GI foods. So you may be a little confused about whether you can eat high GI fruits or vegetables while on the cabbage soup diet. Contrary to earlier belief, the answer nowadays is yes. There is no reason why you can't enjoy a range of fruit such as melons, pineapples, mangos, papaws and many other high GI fruits while on the cabbage soup diet!

When you eat different types of food, your blood sugar level rises at different rates. The food that raises blood sugar the highest is pure table sugar. So the Glycemic Index is a ratio of how high a food raises blood sugar in comparison to how high table sugar raises blood sugar levels. Foods which hold complex carbohydrates that break down and release glucose into the bloodstream slowly cause the blood sugar level to rise steadily and slowly, these foods therefore have low GI scores. Those that have simple carbohydrates break down quickly, causing a rapid, high rise in blood sugar and these have a high GI.

Most beans, whole grains and non-starchy vegetables have a low GI; while sugar, flour made from refined grains, some fruits and root vegetables have a high GI.

If you look at Glycemic Index food lists, then you will see things that should bother an intelligent person. A carrot has almost the same Glycemic Index as sugar does, which seems ridiculous. We all know that a carrot is far safer for diabetics than table sugar. So nutrition scientists developed a new measure to rank foods called Glycemic Load. This tells you how much sugar is in the food, rather than just how high it raises blood sugar levels. To calculate Glycemic Load, you multiply the grams of carbohydrate in a serving of food by that food's Glycemic Index.

Glycemic Load = Grams of Carbohydrate x GI

Carrots and melons both have a high Glycemic Index (GI), but using the new Glycemic Load (GL), carrots (per 120 g serving each) dropped from a higher GI of 47 to a GL of 3.5, while watermelon falls from a GI of 72 to a GL of 4.

The Bottom Line: Foods that are mostly water or air will not cause a steep rise in your blood sugar even if their GI is high. That's why the new measure, Glycemic Load, is more useful when considering your food choices. You can use this knowledge throughout the cabbage soup diet week and also afterwards.

What does this mean for you? If you don't go overboard, then you can of course have high Glycemic fruits and vegetables - even during your diet week. Many of these in small quantities have a safe GL. You can find out more about this important aspect in chapter six. A link to an international table for the Glycemic Index and Glycemic Load can be found in my resource center:
www.successful-diet-cabbage-soup.com/resource-center.html

Ten golden rules for better results

When you are dieting it pays to leave nothing to chance. The Cabbage Soup Diet is hard to go wrong with as long as you follow the diet rules precisely. Here are the ten golden rules for getting your body into "weight loss mode".

1. Get your doctor's permission

This is an important rule for all dieters. I covered this rule in the first chapter and I'm repeating it here because it is so important. Be sure to explain to your doctor that the diet is seven days long. This is a fast weight loss regime and certain medical conditions may make this an unsuitable choice for you. While discussing the matter with your doctor, show them the protein powder you plan to use and check that this is an acceptable option also.

2. Cabbage à la carte

Cook yourself a big pot of cabbage soup - one that lasts all two days. You can vary the recipes according to your taste and make the diet 'your own'. To get you started, you'll find delicious and easy cabbage soup recipes in chapter four.

3. Eat as much cabbage soup as you want!

Once you're started, you can eat cabbage soup as much as you want and whenever you want! In the afternoon, in the evening, as snack… whenever you like! Generally, I wouldn't recommend eating after 6pm when managing or losing weight – but with the cabbage soup I'm making an exception. You can even eat it just before you go to bed if you like.

The more cabbage soup you consume - the better the fat burning and weight loss effect. After preparing the soup, you can store it in your fridge ready to heat and eat whenever you like.

4. Stick to the program

Once you get started, it's really important that you don't make any changes to the order of the program and food. Each step of the diet and the food selected are placed in this special order with the aim of balancing out your insulin levels throughout the week. Stick to this order to achieve the impressive, motivating weight loss you desire!

5. Eat More Slowly

There are a growing number of studies that confirm that by eating slower you'll consume fewer calories. The reason for this is that it takes about 20 minutes for our brains to register that we're full. When we eat fast, we are more likely to continue eating past the point where we're full. By eating slowly, we give our bodies time to realize we're full and stop eating at that point.

6. Drinking!

Do you believe that you need eight glasses (220 ml/7.5 oz) to about 2 liters
(2.1 quarts) of water? While drinking plenty of water is important, when you have excess weight, you should aim to drink another eight glasses for every 20 pounds of additional weight you're carrying. You should also increase your intake of water if you exercise often or live in a hot climate. I recommend spreading out this water consumption

throughout your day. Try to make four or five points in times during your day when you drink a large glass of water, then sip water in between. The most important thing is to never let yourself become thirsty.

Do you hate water or think the taste is yucky? If you feel this way, it is important to understand that drinking other fluids will help hydrate your body, but they are likely to contain additional calories, additives, sugar and other things you don't need. Instead, try adding a slice of lemon to the glass of water, or try fruit or herbal teas.

7. Use a thermos bottle on the road

If you spend a lot of time on the road or you have a hectic schedule, then that's no problem. You can put your cabbage soup in a thermos bottle and take it with you to your office or while you're in the field with your work.

8. Drink Protein Shakes

Don't forget to drink your protein shakes. You'll need to drink two protein shakes per day: One in the morning, the other in the evening. You need this protein to burn fat or you risk your body taking from its own protein reserves, your muscle mass. Organize a good protein powder from a drugstore or check my protein shake recommendation in chapter 3.

9. Vitamins and Minerals

Vitamins and minerals help the body lose fat. If they are missing in your diet, then fat will stay on your hips. Don't worry that you aren't getting these essentials with the Cabbage Soup Diet, as this diet is packed with nutritious vegetables and fruits. To help make doubly sure, it is worthwhile buying a good multivitamin in your drugstore.

Note: If you use my recommended Protein Shake in chapter 3, then you won't need any additional vitamins or minerals as they are already included in the protein shake.

10. Workouts

I can't stress enough the importance of regular exercising to support weight loss. Incorporating regular exercise into your daily life for at least 30 minutes a day will boost your success. If you're unused to exercise then start at a slow pace and build up. Remember, regular physical exercise is just as important for overall health and disease resistance as a healthy, nutritious diet.

7 days and END!

It is important that you only remain on the Cabbage Soup Diet for one week at a time. The diet is relatively low in complex carbohydrates, proteins, vitamins and minerals, which means that prolonged dieting according to this plan could be detrimental to your health. In fact, if you wish to lose only a little weight, then you may find that three days on the Cabbage Soup Diet is enough for you.

With the impressive results and weight loss experienced on the Cabbage Soup Diet you might be tempted to repeat this success the next week. DON'T DO THIS! Use the week's fantastic mind power instead to think about your future nutrition and the improved health and long term benefits of keeping the weight off.

After 7 days you should find that the pounds have melted away. Your body and mind will be more prepared than they've ever been to help you continue losing weight. You'll be ready to make more sensible food choices and maintain your weight loss for the long haul. I've provided some effective suggestions to help you with this in chapter five and six.

The best day to start with your cabbage soup diet

Are you wondering just what the ideal time is to jump start your weight loss? (Hint, it's not when your partner is asking you to lose weight! ;-). The ideal time to lose weight can be any time, but the most important thing is that it is your own free decision. Once you have made that decision, it can be helpful to set aside a quiet week with few social activities while you're on the diet. Look ahead in your diary for a 7 day period, that's party and celebration free and fix that time for dieting!

Starting your diet over Thanksgiving or Christmas is never a good idea however, many readers of my website in the past have found the beginning of the new year is a good opportunity to start the Cabbage Soup Diet.

When I started my first cabbage soup diet I began on a weekend. By choosing the end of the week I was able to have plenty of free time for aerobic exercises and starting my fat burning routine.

Make a clean sweep of all junk food

Carry out a clean sweep of all junk food about 3 days before you start the Cabbage Soup Diet. This 'cold-turkey' method is crucial in the beginning of your **weight loss plan**. By clearing away your junk food from your fridge and cupboards you'll start to free yourself of the cravings and temptation to eat junk food, reducing the chances of breaking the diet. One last important point - Please don't fall in the trap of eating all your junk food in the days before you start the diet!

If you can't bear the thought of wasting food, then why not prepare a food gift basket? You can give away the food to someone who has NO weight problems. You're then ready to start filling your cupboards and refrigerator with fresh fruits and vegetables instead.

Prepare a shopping list ahead of time

Similar to other projects you may take on - success depends upon preparing a good plan and a checklist. Before starting the Cabbage Soup Diet it's always a good idea to write a shopping list. Plan what you're going to eat for the day and if possible, for the week.

Choose your favorite cabbage soup recipe from chapter 4 and note the ingredients for your first cabbage soup. Buy them one day BEFORE you start with your diet, so you avoid temptation in food stores once you start those crucial first days. A great help and time saver is the Cabbage Soup Diet 2.0 shopping list, which you received from me as bonus with this book.
You can shop again if necessary on day 3 or 4, so that you have enough to finish the diet.

Dealing with Family and Friends

Before you begin, work out who you should tell. If you know that a particular friend will be very negative, decide in advance whether he or she really needs to know. (Likewise, telling a supportive friend or family member could be a real bonus during that time.)

If you have a family, then you'll need to consider how to handle family meals. The biggest challenge for you and your family will be days one, two, three and four. By being creative, you can avoid the need to cook separately for yourself and for your family. A great idea is to add filled pasta or shrimps to the basic cabbage soup recipe to make a **satisfying one-pot meal** for your family – not for you! With a bit of forethought, you'll find it easy to incorporate part of your diet plan in your family's meals and simply extend their meals with side dishes like potatoes, pasta or rice.

Don't forget to keep a sense of humor throughout your diet. Remember, your friends and family mean well. Be patient - this is new to them. It can be worthwhile to stay clear of the subject when possible and don't go out of your way to boast about your new lifestyle. Be firm in your decision and remember, it's your decision and your body. Other people may have their opinions, but that's all that they are.

Safe foods that let you "cheat" and not have to worry about

To help you get over any hurdles or urges to snack, I've included a list of 'safe' foods here that let you "cheat". These are all foods you can have without worrying about interfering with the weight loss process. This is a fundamental list, that can help you massively both during and after your diet week. Please don't forget that these are only cheating OPTIONS in case special food cravings occur. You don't have to eat these foods/beverages if you don't need them to help you stick to the diet throughout the week.

1 cup of bran per day

You can have 1 cup of bran per day as a special cheating option. This can really help those who miss something crunchy for breakfast.

Choose only low fat bran which is sugar-free. You can get this from Superstores or check out my resource center for recommendations: www.successful-diet-cabbage-soup.com/resource-center.html

1 flat tablespoon of pumpkin seeds per day

Purchase the pumpkin seeds that are unsalted and unshelled. Measure out 1 tablespoon per day (flat!) and stick to it. Chew these slowly when hunger occurs or drop some over your cabbage soup or salad for variation. You'll find that it takes a long while to eat just one serving of seeds, so it can last throughout the day to help knock out any cravings.

Pumpkin Seeds have several great advantages: aside from the fact that it takes a long time to consume them, they're also very healthy. Pumpkin seeds are packed with zinc, iron, potassium, folic acid and dietary fiber - And last, but not least, they taste delicious!

Please don't eat more than the recommended quantity per day as seeds have one weakness during your diet week. The fat content in the seeds is high, and although the fat is the healthy unsaturated kind, it is still fat that adds to your daily fat consumption.

Cranberry juice is allowed

This is an old cheat and there are several cabbage soup diet plans that allow cranberry juice.

I endorse cranberry juice too (without added sugar), as it has a very low sugar content. Although cranberry juice has a medium glycemic index, it's usually too sour to consume in large quantities.

The 3 biggest traps, you should be prepared for as dieter

Avoid these traps and nothing should stop you from finishing the Cabbage Soup Diet 2.0.

Trap 1: Alcohol

I'm often asked in my forum what kind of alcohol is allowed during the cabbage soup diet week. There are many individuals who think that wine based on fruits like grapes shouldn't be a problem...

To remain clear from the very beginning - NO alcohol is allowed on the Cabbage Soup Diet. If you cheat with alcohol you will jeopardize your weight loss success - and the problem with alcoholic beverages is threefold:

First of all, alcohol almost always leads to overeating and you will set the stage for binge eating. At only two drinks, your body starts craving for more satisfying foods, with yet more calories - making it a diet disaster! Secondly, alcohol contains almost double the calorie content of any type of soda, juice or mixer. And thirdly, one alcoholic drink nearly always leads to more drinks...

Trap 2: Easy access to junk food

Many people are *hypersensitive* when it comes to foods that have high concentrations of fat, sugar, and salt. These people have to overcome years of bad habits and, more difficult still, the physiological reaction that occurs which creates an overwhelming desire to eat these things. Sadly, these habits are hard to shake and the junk food industry has been exploiting this to boost sales. With the powerful persuasion of advertising and the development of such strong cravings for fatty, sugar foods - it's not surprising that a great number of people have to really fight to get rid of these bad habits.

Here comes the trap - if you forget to get rid of the sugary, fatty, salty junk foods in the cupboards or refrigerator BEFORE you start the cabbage soup diet - you'll end up succumbing to temptation. Those foods will be there ready to trip you up, making it incredibly difficult to finish the whole diet week.

For some people, junk food is an addiction - but a little cheating 'fix' with junk food doesn't satisfy them for long. The craving gets stronger, until the desire to eat the whole package (for example, the whole bar of chocolate or box of cookies) is overwhelming. This sense of craving becomes even more heightened while dieting, especially when that food is right in front of them.

The solution: Get rid of temptation - and get rid of ALL of your junk food before you start your diet week!

Trap 3: Restaurants

If you find you have an unexpected invitation to a restaurant and you think that means the end of the diet week - that doesn't have to be so! Depending on your Cabbage Soup Diet day you can always order a lean steak or fish with steamed vegetables or a delicious salad.

In case of the salad, simply request the vinegar-oil-dressing separately or on the side and don't put more than 1 tablespoon dressing over your salad. You can enjoy the meal without even having to admit that you're on a diet, just be prepared before you arrive at the restaurant and you should manage without a hitch!

Chapter 3: Reduce any side effects during the Cabbage Soup Diet 2.0 - Or avoid them all together!

The evolution of the Cabbage Soup Diet 2.0

Now that you've read the basics of the diet, you're probably eagerly awaiting the exact diet plan. Before we start getting into the specifics, it's important that you understand the evolution process of the Cabbage Soup Diet 2.0. By explaining this process, I'm going to present you with the single element that makes this diet faster, safer and easier than you ever imagined.

The prototype Cabbage Soup Diet was incredibly successful at addressing weight loss problems, however there was, and always is, room for improvement. The classic diet was missing one vital element to ensure your health - Protein. The first examples of this diet left the body without this for too long - and going without feeding your body protein can be dangerous.

Over the years, different diet plans were developed, however this lack of protein was never addressed fully. It's most likely that individual dieters put their own spin on the basic plan to compensate for this. The first crucial improvement which started addressing this issue came about at the end of the nineties, when different cabbage soup diet plans incorporated skim milk or low-fat yoghurt as a protein source. Book authors Margret Danbrot (The New Cabbage Soup Diet) and Madeline Cooper (The Ultimate Cabbage Soup Diet), both recommended the daily intake of low fat milk or yoghurt in their diet plans.

Many of my readers who tried these improved diet plans reported amazing results. However there were still a number of my readers who couldn't finish this kind of diet. The hunger was driving them crazy.

At the beginning of the new millennium I stumbled upon a convenient German cabbage soup diet plan which added protein shakes for the first time. I, together with my friends, tried this diet. We were overwhelmed by the impressive results. Over the following years I refined the cabbage soup diet plan, giving it my own spin. In 2004, I published this new plan for the first time **via my website** – www.successful-diet-cabbage-soup.com.

Since then, I've reached thousands of people day per day, helping a great many of them to achieve fantastic results. Along the way, I gained a new found passion about the health of dieters and how to manage it with this convenient cabbage soup diet plan. My diet concept seems to work even better than those with added dairy - as the protein shakes reduce hunger cravings in a far more effective way.

Although the success rate was higher than before – there were still some individuals writing to me seeking advice on how to avoid giving up when they couldn't get over the 2 day hump. So I started researching again, as I wanted to help these people too.

Pushing the envelope

One question that was asked over and over again on my forum was what kind of protein shake I recommend. At the time I had no particular preference. My general recommendation was to use soy protein powder – regardless of brand or type. I also felt back then that soy, whey or any other good quality protein powder would do the job – I believed this from my experience.

All of this changed the day my husband introduced to me a special protein powder that seemed to be a kind of "Jack of all trades". This powder promised to turn your body into a lean, healthy, energy-making, fat-burning machine. As you can imagine - I was electrified!

Now I urge you to read the following closely, this is information you won't find on my website yet. What I'm about to share is what you have all been asking for. I'm going to share with you one of the best protein sources around. This actually makes the convenient Cabbage Soup Diet work even more efficiently. This is just what you need to help you lose weight, burn fat, feel energized, improve your health and look and feel younger.

The <u>ultimate</u> protein shake - a metabolism booster

So now let me present to you the ultimate protein shake for the Cabbage Soup Diet. It's called Almased. This protein shake is genius… It not only boosts your energy - it also preserves your muscle mass.

This shake, alongside the soup, is the single most essential element for success. To help you understanding more about this, I'm including some extract of the theses from German professors Dr. Aloys Berg (university hospital, Freiburg) and Dr. Dr. Ulrich Borchard (Heinrich Heine University, Düsseldorf) - following their studies of Almased.

Here is what they have determined:

1. Almased helps to significantly lower an elevated insulin level, in turn accelerating fat reduction and curbing fat storage.

2. **Almased helps to lower ghrelin[1] levels for a sustained decrease in appetite.**

3. **Almased has a favorable effect regarding the relation between fat and muscle mass. When** accompanied **by routine fitness exercises, it significantly reduces fat pads in the tummy and hip area.**

The protein mix in Almased also activates and stimulates the metabolism in such a way that the body receives the minimum amount it needs to survive and hence, prevents it from synthesizing its own protein. Too much introduced protein in the diet will lead to the formation of deposits on the arterial wall, hence the correct balance is vital. This balance can be found in Almased.

Almased contains pure soybean protein, skim milk yogurt powder and honey. From the inclusion of these basic ingredients in Almased to the way it is produced, every step ensures that the body will be able to absorb the protein efficiently. No low quality soybean flours are used, only produce of the highest quality.

Suggested Use:
To supplement the Cabbage Soup Diet, the following mix is recommended for one protein shake:

1 cup of skim milk (220 ml/7.5 oz) +
3 piled tablespoons of Almased protein powder (35 g/1.23 oz)
If you can't drink milk, you can use water as the liquid base instead

You can have 2 shakes per day while on the diet.
I advise you to make Almased fresh and have it immediately after mixing for best results.

I absolutely love this revolutionary protein supplement. Almased is refreshing and has a palatable, slightly nutty taste. Best of all you

---

[1] **The ghrelin hormone not only stimulates the brain giving rise to an increase in appetite, but also favors the accumulation of lipids in visceral fatty tissue, located in the abdominal zone and considered to be the most harmful. This is the conclusion of research undertaken at Metabolic Research Laboratory of the University Hospital of Navarra, published recently in the International Journal of Obesity.**

don't have to worry about jitters any longer and you never feel really hungry, even while dieting.

One container of Almased (500 g/17.6 oz) is sufficient for the duration of the Cabbage Soup Diet 2.0 week - and costs just $21.95 USD online. If you're serious about getting results as cabbage soup dieter - this is the best investment you can make!

More information about Almased you'll find in my resource center: www.successful-diet-cabbage-soup.com/resource-center.html

Safety on the Cabbage Soup Diet

I've promised you, you won't have to worry when you follow the step by step techniques in my Cabbage Soup Diet 2.0 guide. This diet is low in fat, high in fiber and safe, unlike some high-protein diets. This diet has been around for many years and over that time, the safety of the diet has been improved upon. Now, with the Almased protein shake, this diet is truly safer than ever. So why is it so effective?

Almased is a great choice of protein shake as it contains all the essential amino acids our body requires on a daily basis, plus it holds enzymes that are vital for a healthy metabolism. A new type of technique has allowed the production of the Almased to occur while ensuring vital nutrients retain the most whole, natural form possible. Further to this, Almased has everything you need to achieve genuinely good health. In particular, this shake has a high calcium content, which plays an important role in weight loss, as I'll explain later.

Here are some important facts about protein and Almased:

Fact: Protein is essential for building muscle in your body. In order to ensure your body can build and maintain muscle, you must have a regular supply of easily digested protein.

Fact: In many protein supplements on the market, only about 1/5 of the protein available is likely to present in the bloodstream a few hours after being consumed. If these supplements are not delivering what they promise, then you're not going to have the nutritional benefit, which means you won't see the results you are hoping for.

Fact: The use of Almased, a completely new and highly effective formulation (German patent No. DE AL2 853 194), means that 90% of the amino acids (protein) will be absorbed and evident in your system after just 20 minutes.

Bottom line: The incorporation of the Almased protein shake ensures that you can safely finish the Cabbage Soup Diet <u>without</u> jeopardizing your health.

Getting past the Day 2 hump

I've noted over the years that even experienced cabbage soup dieters have trouble getting past day two, no matter what kind of plan they choose. Getting past the first two days is crucial to your success. The Cabbage Soup Diet 2.0 in combination with Almased protein makes a big difference. You'll find your body now comfortably adapts to the Cabbage Soup Diet.

While day one with fruits is a breeze for most dieters - day two which is based on vegetables gives many a hard time. Understanding this fact BEFORE starting the program makes it easier for you to overcome this challenge. Until now only vegetables were allowed for breakfast on day two. This was tough for many dieters and I can well understand this.

There is a solution: With the Cabbage Soup Diet 2.0, you can now start Day 2 with the Almased Protein Shake and use it as a replacement for breakfast. Many people find the refreshing flavor of the plain protein shake far easier to stomach first thing in the morning.

Here's what happens: When you have the shake for breakfast, it provides you with plenty of energy, puts you in high spirits and keeps you satiated for up to four hours. This change to the diet on day 2 makes it a no-brainer. You'll find it much easier to get through the day and you can have your second protein shake in the evening (1 hour before going to bed).

This change of timing for the protein intake, beside the specific protein recommendation, is the main difference between the convenient cabbage soup diet plan and the Cabbage Soup Diet 2.0. Instead of having the protein shake mid-morning and in the afternoon - you'll now start and end the day with an Almased protein shake.

Using this strategy you still have all the benefits of the successful cabbage soup diet - without the previous plan's breakfast frustrations.

In the report, "Diet with Obesity", researcher Dr. Klosa writes about the unique formulation of Almased. The paper highlights Almased's ability to reduce hunger in a totally natural way. The benefit of this for the dieter is that this relieves any problems of tiredness and irritability that frequently occur when using other weight loss programs.

Coffee and Dieting

Before I begin going through each day in detail, let me explain my thoughts on coffee and dieting. You will see in the plan that for drinks I recommend herbal or fruit teas and water, no coffee! Although several cabbage soup diet plans allow coffee I don't really recommend it for successful weight loss. Here's why:

Some facts about coffee

While most people wouldn't view something as typical to the American way of life as coffee as a "drug", there are certain properties of this beverage that are drug-like:

• Caffeine is a stimulant.
• It can change your mood.
• It is addictive.

And - unfortunately- it's bad for losing weight! There are two main reasons why coffee can be a problem for you when you're trying to drop the pounds. One reason is physiological and the other is psychological.

Physiological

Coffee excites the adrenal glands which produce stress hormones. A steady attack on these glands from sugar, coffee, daily life and stress, can cause "adrenal exhaustion". Coffee can destroy your optimal blood sugar balance. The body reacts to coffee as a jolt or "stress response", much like the adrenals shooting adrenaline into the system. Hence, coffee is a signal for the release of sugar. What usually follows is several hours of jitteriness and a drop in your blood sugar level. Before you know it you're burning, crashing and reaching for... you guessed it - sugary snacks!

Psychological

The psychological effects occur because coffee perfectly matches the receptors for adenosine - a brain chemical that is partly responsible for keeping you calm.

In effect, coffee switches off the adenosine, making you feel 'wired' and awake. While there are some situations where people find this attribute of coffee useful, this added nervousness and stimulation creating jumpiness exactly when feeling calm would be an advantage is not a good thing. Combine the psychological effects with the physiological blood sugar fluctuations and you can end up with enormous hunger cravings. *Not* the best state for a successful diet week.

My recommendation: If you cannot get by without it, then drink unsweetened coffee only when absolutely necessary. While 2-3 cups of black, sugar free coffee per day is ok while on the cabbage soup diet, ultimately, the diet week will be much easier without coffee.

Note: The Cabbage Soup Diet is much lower in fat and calories than your regular diet, so the caffeine in coffee or black tea may have a greater influence on your body than it would otherwise. This might also result in increased feelings of stress and tension.

The solution: If you're able to replace coffee with a natural fat burner like green tea, then you'll find this can be very therapeutic. Having green tea alongside every meal is a sure fire way to boost your weight loss. The tea contains just 4 calories per serving - plus it is a metabolic stimulant. Drinking green tea without any additives will ensure you get the most benefit from this beverage. The tea will increase body function and help burn even more calories. Added to that, the polyphenols in this beverage aid in the digestion of fats - making it an all round winner!

So now that I've covered all the essentials that go hand in hand with this diet - let's have a look at the actual diet itself:

The Cabbage Soup Diet 2.0 plan overview

Diet Day	Cabbage Soup Diet 2.0
Day One:	Cabbage soup Fruits except bananas 2 Almased protein shakes Water with lemon, herbal or fruit teas
Day Two:	Cabbage soup Vegetables , For dinner - a big baked potato with butter 2 Almased protein shakes Water with lemon, herbal or fruit teas
Day Three:	Cabbage soup Fruits (except bananas) and vegetables 2 Almased protein shakes Water with lemon, herbal or fruit teas
Day Four:	Cabbage soup 3 – 6 bananas, Low fat milk/yoghurt 2 Almased protein shakes Water with lemon, herbal or fruit teas
Day Five:	Cabbage soup Poultry or fish, Tomatoes 2 Almased protein shakes Water with lemon, herbal or fruit teas
Day Six:	Cabbage soup Poultry or fish, Vegetables 2 Almased protein shakes Water with lemon, herbal or fruit teas
Day Seven:	Cabbage soup Brown rice, Vegetables 2 Almased protein shakes Water with lemon, herbal or fruit teas

On the following pages, I've put together an exact, foolproof Cabbage Soup Diet 2.0 plan. This gives you suggestions for each day based upon the outline on the previous page. Using the following day by day plan should help make completing the Cabbage Soup Diet 2.0 week as easy and successful as possible.

Day 1 - Fruit Day

DAY 1	FRUIT DAY
Overview	Welcome to your first day of the Cabbage Soup Diet 2.0 week. The first day is a straightforward one, where you can eat as many fruits as you want except for bananas. For drinks, choose water with lemon or herbal or fruit teas.
Breakfast	Mix 1 cup of skim milk (220 ml/7.5 oz) + 3 piled tablespoons of Almased Protein Powder (35 g/1.23 oz)
Breaktime	Have a fruity 'second breakfast' using any fruits that take your fancy. I recommend you to choose the freshest, seasonal fruits from your region.
Lunch	Eat one portion of cabbage soup (or two or three ...) And of course, you may add as many fruits as you like to your lunch.
Afternoon Break	If you want you can prepare yourself a big bowl of fruit salad. *Hint* - Add extra taste to the fruit salad with squeezed lemon juice (rich in vitamin C).
Dinner	Start with a bowl of cabbage soup and then enjoy some more fruit if you feel like them. Try to have dinner early and avoid eating fruit after 6 pm as they may be too much for your digestive system.
In the evening (1 hour before bedtime at the latest)	Mix 1 cup of skim milk (220 ml/7.5 oz) + 3 piled tablespoons of Almased Protein Powder (35 g/1.23 oz).

Tips for Day 1

If you find at any stage between the portions recommended that hunger is overwhelming, simply go to your fridge and heat up a portion of cabbage soup. I like mine really hot and I find it simple to just heat in my microwave. There is also plenty of evidence to suggest that hot soups are more satisfying, helping to get rid of hunger and make you feel more comfortable and relaxed. You can eat as much soup as you want and you can even have hot soup to fill and relax you just before going to bed.

Allowed fruits on Day 1

The following list is some of the best fruits for the diet in alphabetical order:
Apples, apricots, blackberries, blueberries, (bing) cherries, grapefruits, grapes, kiwifruits, mangos, nectarines, peaches, pears, plums, oranges, pawpaws, raspberries, strawberries, tangerines...I'm sure you'll find many more and fresh seasonal fruits have many additional health benefits.

Tip: On hot summer days, I mix some frozen fruit and cranberry juice in a blender for a terrific fruit slushie.

"Fluid Fruits"

If you don't like fruit that much, then it can help to change consistency. Cut fruit into very small pieces, shred it or mix up a fruit smoothie or make fresh squeezed juice. The key is not to go overboard on fruit juices in place of fresh, whole fruit, as you will reduce the effectiveness of the diet.

In particular, premade fruit juice in bottles could leave you very hungry as the satiation effect of fruit juice is not as high as when you eat the whole fruit. Bottled juices pass through your system faster and on top of that they influence your insulin level in a negative way.

Why you must avoid dried fruits

The problem with dried fruit is that the drying process means that all the sugar is retained while all the water is removed. When you compare dried fruit to fresh fruit, it is very high in calories and this makes it unsuitable for those trying to lose weight.

On top of this, dried fruit not only has a high Glycemic Index, but in most instances (e.g. figs, raisins), it also has a high Glycemic Load - which indicates that it is a food type to be avoided, otherwise you risk getting very hungry...

Want an example of how this works? In one cup of raisins, you'll find the same number of calories as a pound of grapes. That means that 1 cup of raisins contains 500 calories, while 1 cup of grapes contains only 70 calories –a big difference! Another thing to consider is that the fiber in dried fruit is less successful in satisfying your hunger.

So even after completing the cabbage soup diet, dried fruits should only be consumed in small quantities.

What about canned or preserved fruits?

These are a no go as well. These fruits will usually contain added sugar to preserve the fruit. NEVER get fruits that have been kept in syrup. They are much better if they have been kept in natural juices. Even those with natural juice aren't the best choice when you are on the fruit days - it is possible for loss of vitamin C to occur during the canning process.

Day 2 - Vegetable Day

DAY 2	VEGETABLE DAY
Overview	On your second day you can stuff yourself with all the vegetables you can eat. That means all the raw, steamed or cooked vegetables of your choice. You are literally free to eat all the vegetables you want alongside the regular cabbage soup. When eating these things, make sure you stay away from legumes like beans, pulses, peas or corn. At dinner, you can reward yourself with a big baked potato with butter. There are no fruits allowed on Day 2.
Breakfast	Mix 1 cup of skim milk (220 ml/7.5 oz) + 3 piled tablespoons of Almased Protein Powder (35 g/1.23 oz)
Breaktime	Vegetables: cut carrots, radish, cucumber, pepper and fennel in small pieces - slicing or shredding some for variety. I recommend seasonal vegetables from your region, which will mean they are freshest and full of nutrients. If you're not ready for vegetables, then you might want to have a bowl of cabbage soup instead.
Lunch	Vegetables in the Wok: Directions: Heat 1 teaspoon olive oil in a coated wok or pan. Put in vegetables, cut in small pieces - e.g. carrots, scallions, leek, cabbage and chinese cabbage. Cook rapidly in the wok until the vegetables are firm to the bite. Season to taste with pepper, herbs and 1 teaspoon of soy sauce. To make sure you feel full through the afternoon, have a bowl of cabbage soup or a salad as a starter.
Afternoon Break	Vegetables/cabbage soup
Dinner	A bowl of hot cabbage soup & one big baked potato. Directions: Wrap a big potato in aluminum foil, bake it for 75 - 90 minutes at 440 F (225 degrees) (alternative: 3 cooked small potatoes in the skin.) Eat the potatoes with some butter (1 teaspoon) or low fat white cheese (3 tablespoons).
In the evening	Mix 1 cup of skim milk (220 ml/7.5 oz) + 3 piled tablespoons of Almased Protein Powder (35 g/1.23 oz)

Tips for Day 2

Most dieters (me included), find day 2 the most challenging day of the diet week. This is the most restrictive day of the diet as far as food choices go, however with the Almased protein this shouldn't be a problem anymore.

List of Vegetables

Here is a list of allowed vegetables/herbs/roots for the vegetable days. Use these kind of vegetables also as variation for your cabbage soup: Artichoke, Asparagus, Aubergine, Beetroot, Egg plant, Broccoli, (White) Cabbage, Cauliflower, Carrots, Celery, Chili, Cucumber, Fennel, Garlic, Kohlrabi, Leek, Lettuce, Mushroom, Onions, Parsley, Pepper/Capsicum, Pumpkin, Radish, Spinach, Spring onion, Squash, Tomatoes, (Brussels) Sprouts, Zucchini /Courgette

Not allowed: avocados, legumes, corn, soy beans, beans, pulses, lentils

Keep in mind, that Day 2 is the day where you should add a variety of intense and pleasing flavors so that you can have plenty of variety to help keep those hunger pains at bay!

Nibble Carrots

Are you feeling nervous and lacking concentration? It could be because your brain is really feeling the impact of your change in diet. No problem: Nibble carrots. These vegetables can help to supply the necessary "natural sweetness" that your brain needs to regain focus!

No avocados!

Avocados are not accepted as a suitable vegetable for the vegetable days because of their high fat content. Avocados are very healthy, but they are also one of the vegetables with the highest fat content. Even after the diet week I recommend you eat this vegetable only in limited quantities to maintain your weight loss.

Salad Dressing

You may have 1 tablespoon healthy (olive) oil throughout the day, plus 1 tablespoon of vinegar per day while on cabbage soup diet.

Combining these ingredients can build a great salad dressing, so you don't have to worry that it might be a little bland. Usually for one salad portion, one teaspoon of oil and one of vinegar is enough. If you are not sure that you want vinegar, then try lemon juice for a great alternative.

Note: Don't consume more than 1 tablespoon (olive) oil per day. No other sauces! The remaining (olive) oil can be used to sauté some vegetables for your cabbage soup or a delicious vegetable dish.

Day 3 - Fruit and Vegetable Day

DAY 3	FRUIT AND VEGETABLE DAY
Overview	Congratulations! You've passed the 2 day hump. Knowing that you've overcome the hardest day of the diet week should give you a big confidence boost and added motivation for the rest of the week. With the first two days out of the way, it gets easier here on in…
	Day 3 is one of my favorite days. Why? Because you have a choice between almost all the fruits and vegetables. That means you have a lot of flexibility in preparing your meals. Mix up some ideas from Day 1 and Day 2: Eat all the soup, fruits and vegetables you want, except for the potato. Don't forget to drink at least eight big glasses/cups of water with lemon, herbal or fruit teas.
	No bananas today!
Breakfast	Mix 1 cup of skim milk (220 ml/7.5 oz) + 3 piled tablespoons of Almased Protein Powder (35 g/1.23 oz)
Breaktime	Fruits or vegetables.
Lunch	For lunch a big bowl of cabbage soup. If you wish, you can have a salad as starter. Of course, you may also have additional fruits and vegetables for lunch if you like.
Afternoon Break	Fruits or vegetables.
Dinner	Cabbage Soup and more fruits, salad or vegetables. All together or one by one, whatever you like and prefer. Don't forget to vary your preparation for added interest: Try preparing in a bowl, foil, grilled or steamed in a wok...
In the evening	Mix 1 cup of skim milk (220 ml/7.5 oz) + 3 piled tablespoons of Almased Protein Powder (35 g/1.23 oz)

Tips for Day 3

Avoid problems at the office

If you're working while doing the diet, take some fruits and vegetables cut in stripes with you. You should also take a big thermos bottle with the magic soup. The more soup you eat the better. And maybe your colleagues want to taste your wonderful soup too...

Canteen or Restaurant Tips

In case you want to have lunch with your colleagues, here are some helpful hints: Eat a portion of cabbage soup before you go, then order a salad with a separate dressing: vinegar, a teaspoon of olive oil, plus a little salt and pepper. Steamed vegetables are also allowed – these are best prepared in a coated pan with just a little olive oil. (In good restaurants this shouldn't be a problem!)

Special Tips for the Fruit and Vegetable Diet Day 3

Why not try some exotic fruits? Papayas and Mangos are a good option, as these contain enzymes that help boost your protein metabolism.

You may also want to prepare a frozen version of any of the allowed fruits and vegetables – as long as it's frozen plain and with no syrup, butter or sauce.

Marinate your exotic salad with orange and lemon juice. For best results avoid sugar or artificial sweeteners.

Day 4 - Banana Day

DAY 4	BANANA DAY
Overview	Day 4 is **banana diet** day. That means it's time to give yourself a pat on the back - you've reached the 'semifinal' and you're attacking your last pounds. You should eat at least 3-4 bowls cabbage soup on this day. For variation you may mix it to a "soup puree" if you like. You'll find you may begin to experience carbohydrate cravings around this time. It's very important that you follow the guidelines for managing this with bananas on this day, as this food choice lessens your desire for sweets and eliminates much of the gassiness the cabbage soup might produce. The main food you'll be eating on day four is bananas and skim milk. You can eat up to six bananas and drink up to eight glasses of skim milk if you like on this day, along with your soup. Don't forget to drink at least eight big glasses of water, herbal or fruit teas.
Breakfast	Mix 1 cup of skim milk (220 ml/7.5 oz) + 3 piled tablespoons of Almased Protein Powder (35 g/1.23 oz)
Breaktime	1 banana shake.
Lunch	For lunch a big bowl of cabbage soup, 1 banana.
Afternoon Break	1 banana shake, cabbage soup.
Dinner	Cabbage Soup and 1 banana. If you want to vary your preparation of the banana: try frying or baking your banana.
In the evening	Mix 1 cup of skim milk (220 ml/7.5 oz) + 3 piled tablespoons of Almased Protein Powder (35 g/1.23 oz)

Tips for Day 4

Tip 1:
You don't need to eat 6 plain bananas, you can preparing some as a shake during the day if you prefer.

Tip 2:

Check your "cabbage soup stock". If you've been having the same soup for several days, you may wish to try out a new variation. You'll find plenty of recipe ideas on my website and in Chapter Four.

Skim milk substitutes

If you don't drink milk, or you want a little more variety, then you may substitute the skim milk for plain natural yoghurt (low fat), butter milk (low fat) or even soy milk. A delicious variation in summer is a banana smoothie based on banana and fat free yogurt with crushed ice.

Possible banana substitutes

Some people can't eat bananas. Just the smell of them makes them feel sick. On the other hand you should ideally consume at least 3 bananas on Day 4. Bananas are high in carbohydrates and calories. They are important because they provide a sweet change of pace and texture from the other food of the diet, while supplying you with vitamin A, iron, niacin, some protein and an abundance of potassium. Your body especially needs the carbohydrates and potassium today.

Pawpaw (papaya) also known as Indian banana, might be a good substitute for bananas, if it's available in your area. You should eat the pawpaw fresh. (Tip: pawpaw is often substituted for bananas when baking banana bread)

If pawpaw is not available in your area, then try apricots or kiwi fruit. From a nutritional viewpoint, apricots, kiwi fruit and pawpaw outrank bananas as the top low-sodium, high-potassium fruits. Kiwi and pawpaw are also fruits that provide high levels of nutrition. The pawpaw is very low in fat - and one of these fruits has just half the calories of a large banana.

Day 5 - Fish & Tomato Day

DAY 5	FISH & TOMATO DAY
Overview	Today, you'll need to eat 10 to 20 oz (300 - 600 g) of fish, plus up to six fresh tomatoes. Drink at least 10 big glasses of water on this day. The water is needed to helps cleanse uric acid from your body. Eat the cabbage soup at least twice during the day - the more often the better. If you prefer poultry or beef, you can substitute lean cuts for the fish. No other vegetables today besides of those in your cabbage soup and also no fruits!
Breakfast	Mix 1 cup of skim milk (220 ml/7.5 oz) + 3 piled tablespoons of Almased Protein Powder (35 g/1.23 oz)
Breaktime	Tomatoes
Lunch	**Tomato Codfish Filet** 150 g codfish filet 3 tomatoes 1 tablespoon torn fresh herbs (like: parsley, chives, dill) 1 chopped or crushed garlic clove 2 teaspoon lemon juice 2 teaspoon olive oil Salt and pepper Directions: 1. Heat the oven to 200° degrees, wash the codfish and dry. Season with lemon juice, salt and pepper. Wash the tomatoes and remove the shaft. Cut into thick pieces. 2. Lightly oil a piece of aluminum foil using olive oil. Place the tomatoes on the foil, add salt and pepper, garlic and herbs. Place the fish on top of that with 1 teaspoon of olive oil. Fold the foil and close it firmly. Bake it for 20 minutes at 200° degrees.
Afternoon Break	Tomatoes/cabbage soup.
Dinner	Cabbage Soup, lean fish or steak with tomato plate.
In the evening	Mix 1 cup of skim milk (220 ml/7.5 oz) + 3 piled tablespoons of Almased Protein Powder (35 g/1.23 oz)

Tips for Day 5

Fatburning Fish!

Fish supplies valuable protein which helps your body to burn fat. Saltwater fish is rich in omega 3 fatty acids, which protect your heart and your nervous system. Fish also provides you with necessary iodine - to help thyroid function and promote the production of active hormones that keep you slim. If you don't normally eat much fish, then after you complete the cabbage soup diet week, you may also find it beneficial to add fish meals to your weekly meal planning.

Would like to try fish on day 5, but you're worried about fish bones? No problem! There are many fish that are almost boneless. Here are some good examples of boneless fish: hake, walleye, bass and sole. Even codfish has almost no bones. Pay attention, however, that your fish is low in fat. For the best results during the diet week I recommend codfish, hake, haddock and plaice.

Tip 1: Shell Fish and Shrimps

Another great option is to use shell fish and shrimps on the fish day. For variation you might also like to add some shrimps to your cabbage soup. The cabbage soup will taste delicious - like a gourmet soup! That's why I make this kind of cabbage soup variation even nowadays.

Tip 2: Tuna Salad

A tuna salad with tomatoes and onions is another great idea for day five. Mix a small tin of tuna preserved in water (without oil) with tomato and onion rings. Sprinkle some vinegar-oil dressing over this delicious combination.

Use skinless poultry

If you prefer poultry on the day 5 then make sure that it is skinless. A great option is to use poultry breast (skinless) and this can also add variation to your cabbage soup.

Directions for tomato plate:

Wash the fresh tomatoes, remove the shaft and cut into slices.
Place it on a plate, drizzle 1-2 teaspoon Aceto Balsamico (Balsamic vinegar) and 1 teaspoon of olive oil over top and garnish with fresh basil leaves.

Wonderful Tomato variations:

A tomato is a fruit from "Paradise" - helping your body by providing lots of potassium to detoxify with. Tomato may also prevent cancer. Here is a great tomato variation that you can use with this diet: Wash fresh tomatoes, remove the shaft and cut in to thick pieces. Puree in a mixer. Season with salt, pepper, 1 teaspoon olive oil and 1 teaspoon vinegar. Garnish with basil leaves. Enjoy it cold as a sauce with your steak or warm it up to have as a soup.

Can I eat fish and chicken in the same day on meat day? Please explain what proteins can be mixed together for best results on the same day?

Yes, you may have all type of lean meat or fish on the meat day. But cut the fat out! There is no perfect combination, but poultry or fish with vegetables for lunch and a big steak with salad for dinner I find works very well. Make sure you limit the amount of salt on the meat.

Are there any allowed sauces to marinate the meat?

For a marinade you may use mustard or soy sauce - however use this in limited quantities. These are high in salt content, so I recommend not to use more than **one tablespoon** per day. Salt retains water in your body and the effect of the cabbage soup diet might be diluted.

Day 6 - Meat Day

DAY 6	MEAT DAY
Overview	Eat poultry and vegetables. You can even have two or three steaks if you like, with vegetables, but no potato. Make sure you eat your soup at least twice, preferably three times during the day. Drink at least eight big glasses of water throughout the day.
Breakfast	Mix 1 cup of skim milk (220 ml/7.5 oz) + 3 piled tablespoons of Almased Protein Powder (35 g/1.23 oz)
Breaktime	Vegetables
Lunch	**Chicken Pan Recipe** 100 g chicken breast fillet 100 g snow peas 1/2 red pepper 2 spring onions 40 g soy sprouts 1 tablespoon soy sauce 3 tablespoon vegetable broth 1 teaspoon oil, Salt and black pepper Directions: Cut chicken breast in thin slices. Mix 1 tablespoon of soy sauce with the pepper, turn your meat in it and let it steep for 5 minutes. Wash the snow peas and cook them for 2 minutes in salt water. Wash your red pepper and cut it into small cubes. Wash the spring onions and cut into fine rings. Wash the sprouts under hot water in a strainer and let them drip dry. Heat a small amount of oil in a coated pan or wok. Stir fry your chicken meat for 3-4 minutes. Remove the cooked chicken from the pan and set aside where it will remain warm. Stir fry your vegetables and sprouts for 4-5 minutes, then pour in the broth and add pepper to taste. Don't forget to have your cabbage soup as a starter! Enjoy your meal!
Afternoon Break	Vegetables/cabbage soup
Dinner	Cabbage soup, lean steak with a vegetable plate
In the evening	Mix 1 cup of skim milk (220 ml/7.5 oz) + 3 piled tablespoons of Almased Protein Powder (35 g/1.23 oz)

Tips for Day 6

For quantity you should eat the same as for the fish day. You may have up to 600 gram (20 oz) lean poultry, fish or beef on each of the "meat days". E.g. 300 gram (10 oz) for lunch and 300 gram (10 oz) for dinner.

Tip 1: Add poultry or fish to your cabbage soup

You can also add some poultry or fish and vegetables to your cabbage soup - as much as you want.

Tip 1: Poultry in the morning

You can eat a piece of skinless poultry in the morning. To help the body accept the protein, add some lemon juice on the poultry.

Directions for the vegetable plate:

Wash and cut a variety of fresh vegetables (such as tomatoes, cucumber, pepper…). Arrange the vegetables on a plate. Drizzle 1-2 teaspoons of vinegar and 1 teaspoon of olive oil over the top and garnish with fresh herb leaves.

Meat Substitution for Vegetarians

Are you a vegetarian? No problem! If you are, you can still make the cabbage soup diet work for you. How? Just replace the meat/chicken meals on day 5 + 6 with tofu meals. Tofu is a vegetarian product based on soy beans with high nutritional value. Many vegetarians appreciate this product for its ability to provide plenty of protein to replace meat.

Tofu is available in all larger supermarkets, as well as in special grocery stores.

You may also like to buy it online - for help with this, see my tofu recommendation in the resource center:
www.successful-diet-cabbage-soup.com/resource-center.html

Below is a low fat tofu recipe suggestion (2 servings) for the "meat days".
This recipe is best prepared in a wok:
1 green or yellow bell pepper, cubed
1 onion, cubed
1/2 pound tofu, cubed
1/2 pound mushrooms, halved
1 teaspoon sunflower oil
1 teaspoon basil
1 teaspoon low sodium seasoning
some pepper

Directions:
In hot oil, sweat onions in a wok. Add mushrooms, tofu, seasoning, water & herbs. Simmer till your vegetables are limp.

You may eat all of the two portions at once eg. for lunch and prepare another "new batch" for dinner. For variation you may wish to exchange vegetables and try it with carrots, zucchini, leek or tomatoes instead of peppers.

Can I have Quorn instead of meat?

Yes, you may have Quorn instead of meat. Quorn is even healthier than the equivalent meat dish, as it is based on mycoprotein, a totally vegetable protein. On top of that, Quorn is also very versatile.
- Day 5: Quorn & tomatoes + cabbage soup
- Day 6: Quorn & all vegetables (no potato) + cabbage soup

Day 7 - Rice Day

DAY 7	RICE DAY
Overview	Day 7 of the diet is based on brown rice and vegetables. Again eat cabbage soup to your heart's content. It is also important that you eat your soup at least three times on this day. Drink at least eight big glasses of water throughout the day.
Breakfast	Mix 1 cup of skim milk (220 ml/7.5 oz) + 3 piled tablespoons of Almased Protein Powder (35 g/1.23 oz)
Breaktime	Vegetables
Lunch	**Risotto with Mushrooms** 1 small onion 3 cloves of garlic 2 carrots 150 g (5.2 oz) champignons or other mushrooms 80 g (2.8 oz) fast cooking natural rice 175 ml (6 oz) hot vegetable broth 1 teaspoon olive oil, 1 teaspoon lemon juice salt, black pepper, 5 branches parsley Directions: Peal the onion and cut into small cubes. Finely chop or crush the cloves of garlic. Heat the oil in a pot and steam the onion and garlic 1-2 minutes. Stir in the rice and fry for about a minute, then add the hot broth. Let it simmer at low heat for 20-25 minutes. Peal the carrots and cut them into thin slices. Wash the mushrooms and cut into thin slices too. After the rice has been simmering for 10 minutes, add both carrots and mushrooms, and continue to stir from time to time. Wash the parsley, dry it and roughly chop the leaves. Add some salt, pepper and lemon juice to the risotto to taste. At the end of the cooking add the chopped parsley.
Afternoon Break	Vegetables/cabbage soup
Dinner	Cabbage soup, lean steak with a vegetable plate
In the evening	Mix 1 cup of skim milk (220 ml/7.5 oz) + 3 piled tablespoons of Almased Protein Powder (35 g/1.23 oz)

Tips for Day 7

Cook yourself your favorite cabbage soup

If your cabbage soup stock has almost run out, then cook yourself another batch of your favorite recipe. Even if you can't eat it all today, you can still freeze the remaining soup for use as a starter before your regular meals the following days. In chapter 5 I'll explain why this is an excellent idea.

How much brown rice can I have on the rice day?

Brown rice is very filling and it's difficult to overeat - especially in combination with sufficient cabbage soup. From my personal experience I wouldn't use more than 100 g (3.5 oz) of uncooked rice - the equivalent of 200g (7 oz) of cooked rice. For the recipe on the rice diet page you need approximately 80 g (2.8 oz) rice.

I know some dieters who ate more than 200 g (7 oz) cooked rice and still had successful weight loss. It depends on the individual too.

Can I use white rice instead of brown rice? Will this change the effects?

Brown and white rice both flush water of your body, which is why you could use both from a weight loss perspective. I recommend however brown or natural rice. Brown rice is healthier and contains more nutrients and fibers. This type of rice has a better influence on your insulin level. It will stabilize insulin levels and reduce the risk of binge eating after completing the 7 day Cabbage Soup Diet 2.0.

If you don't have brown or natural rice, or you can't get it in your region, then you may try completing the diet with white rice. Please be aware that white rice might sometimes mean hunger attacks.

Final Words

You've now completed your last cabbage soup diet day. Congratulations! Maybe you want to reward yourself with a body wrap this evening. I'll tell you more about this in short.

After day 7 your diet is at an end and you can enjoy your life with a better understanding of weight loss and good nutrition.

The biggest lesson I hope you'll come away with is that nutrition is good for you. With the "right" nutrition you'll have more energy, feel more satisfied with your body and you'll feel your spirit revived.

In the following section - I've covered numerous useful tips and hints on how to manage the diet week even more successfully.

Master your cravings in just days - and never rely on willpower alone to lose weight again!

First of all it is important you learn to differentiate between physical cravings (hunger) and psychological cravings. I promised you that you will never feel hungry with the Cabbage Soup Diet 2.0 - now I want to help you stay in control of that hunger always.

Physical Food Cravings (Hunger)

If you feel physical food cravings (hunger), then first thing you should do is to check whether you're dehydrated. The body generally doesn't send the message that you are thirsty until you are on the verge of dehydration. Most often, dehydration occurs as mild hunger, so the first thing to do in that case is to drink a full glass of water. If this doesn't satisfy you then you may like to try the following:

- Have cabbage soup even before bed time
- Make sure you have access to a range of safe foods that allow you to "cheat" (see chapter 2).
- Have plenty of fruits and vegetables on the days they are allowed

Often a small amount of high-carbohydrate food provides enough to ease your hunger. Fruits with higher sugar content can be useful for this on the fruit days. Cravings on the banana day shouldn't be a problem as the banana is high in carbohydrates.

On vegetable days, you may try carrots. Nibbling carrots is a great way to supply your body with the necessary carbohydrates to minimize those blood sugar dips.

Most importantly: The incorporation of the Almased protein shake for breakfast and in the evening makes this diet hunger proof. This shake is so effective you won't have any thoughts of junk food.

Carbohydrate rich foods usually satisfy most dieters experiencing hunger.
Some dieters may still struggle, experiencing cravings no matter how much cabbage soup they consume, free fruits and vegetables they eat, or how many protein shakes they drink.

These dieters may find that they are not truly experiencing physical cravings for food (hunger), but rather an emotional craving. This makes a big difference. The key is to trust yourself to learn to judge whether you crave food for emotional reasons or whether your body is truly hungry.

Psychological Food Cravings (emotional)

An emotional craving presents the following traits:

- You are not genuinely physiologically hungry
- It is not relieved when you try to wait it out (for around ten minutes)
- The craving does not intensify over time; but the emotion does
- Doing something else satisfies the real need, and the craving disappears

If you think you're suffering emotional food cravings, then this is generally due to **boredom** or **lack of fulfillment**.

Cravings Due to Boredom

In case of boredom, the simple answer is to find more interesting things to do. This technique has helped many dieters to achieve success. If you know that you start to experience cravings the minute you sit down to watch TV, then you may find it beneficial to give yourself something extra to do while watching your favorite programs. If you can knit or crochet, or you have some other crafty pastime you enjoy, then that could be the perfect way to take your mind off of the cravings.

When you have nothing to do and you feel a little bored, this is often a trigger for those pesky cravings.

If you want to manage this and avoid that from becoming a problem, then you might try jotting down a few ideas for things to do to avoid the cravings. The next time that you are at a loose end and you have that urge to overeat, get your list out and find something to do until the cravings pass.

Cravings Due to lack of Fulfillment

Lack of fulfillment can arise when you are dissatisfied with a relationship, have an inappropriate exercise routine, are stressed, have an uninspiring job or lack a spiritual practice. Each of these things may all be triggers for emotional eating.

Often this problem occurs when we are trying to fill a void left by a lifestyle that is not nourishing or feeding our needs. Do you have enough sweetness; i.e., joy, fun, laughter or relaxation in your life? If not, then the chances are that you're trying to get those basic needs met with sweet foods. Do you express your emotions in a healthy, assertive way? Cravings for high-fat foods are often a means of calming, even numbing, negative emotional states.

Next time you experience this kind of craving - think about what it is that you're really wanting? Usually it's not the food. Un-met needs can cause cravings. Perhaps it's a need for more sleep, quiet alone time, a more active social life, or a stronger connection with healthy, positive, like-minded people. Prepare a list of your unmet needs and think about how you can take steps to have your basic needs met in healthy ways. Consider which of these needs could be met as a special reward during your diet week – for example, going to a cultural event with your best friend. You may find that consulting a specialized book will help you understand how to overcome a lack of life fulfillment. You can then begin planning how you can tackle these needs in future. Write your thoughts down in your diet journal. There will be more about the diet journal and your reward system in the next section.

If you're willing to do the "inner" work, you'll find that it's not that difficult to satisfy cravings in a healthy, non-food way.

Keeping up motivation during the diet week

Most dieters have some degree of motivation, as they have already decided to take action when they made the decision to do the Cabbage Soup Diet. The biggest problem is keeping up the levels to prevent any relapses during the week. In this section you'll learn how to develop a different mindset, which will increase your desire for success!

Many of the following ideas are based on work done by weight control experts and psychologists. Other tips and suggestions grew out of my own experience and the plain common sense passed on by my engaged readers, who discovered that certain approaches were helpful for them and shared them with the community.

Keep a diet journal

I believe that this is one of the most important motivational tips of all. Your journal will help you keep track of all the facts. For instance you'll record your starting weight and measurements in your diet book. You'll then weigh and measure yourself twice during the diet - On day one and on the morning after you complete day seven. This will help you to evaluate after your seven days how much you've lost in terms of pounds and inches.

For me, my diet journal was more than just a record keeping device. In fact writing in it was a form of self-talk, realized in ink or pencil. This motivating tool reaffirmed my intention to stick to the rules of the diet and cheer myself on.

There may be times during the diet, when you feel a little shaky. Times when cravings occur and you feel tempted to eat a favorite food that's not allowed.

I experienced times when I didn't feel at all positive about the possibility of losing the weight I wanted to lose. Never mind what it is that you experience during the diet. Write what you believe. As with positive self-talk, the strong words and phrases you use in your diet journal will take on a power of their own. Writing good things in your journal is like a self-fulfilling prophecy in a very real sense. In the following section I'll go deeper into how a creative process can help throughout the diet.

The kind of diet journal I'm talking about is different from a diary, in which you confess also your failures and darkest fears.

Just as positive writing has the power to strengthen and motivate you, negative writing can undermine and weaken your resolve.

It can be helpful, however to write about close calls - times when you felt tempted to chuck the diet and go for a high-calorie, chocolate attack. When you didn't succumb and instead determined the kind of craving underlying this urge – whether real hunger or emotional craving - then write down how you overcame this feeling. The fact that you resisted proves how strong and committed you are. That's something to feel positive about and give yourself credit for.

Keeping a food diary can help you identify your most important eating triggers and formulate solutions to overcome them. This will in turn form a valuable pattern for the time after the diet week.

Attract your perfect weight and body using the Creative Process

To achieve your perfect body and ideal weight, you can begin by moving mentally closer to your goal. The following steps have proved to be very successful in that process.

Step 1: Ask

Be clear on the weight you want to be. Have a picture in your mind of what you will look like when you have achieve your perfect weight. If this is a weight you were before, then get pictures of yourself at your perfect weight and reflect upon them often. If you haven't pictures of yourself at your ideal weight, then get some images of the kind of body you would like to have and look at those often.

Step 2: Believe

Belief is a critical element in your success. You must believe you will receive what you wish for and that the perfect weight is yours already. You must imagine, pretend, make-believe and act as if that perfect weight is yours already. You must see yourself as being that perfect weight.

Make sure that your thoughts, words and actions don't conflict with what you ask for. Buying clothes at your current would be one example of this. Instead think on the great clothes you could buy to fit you when you reach your ideal body weight. Think of achieving your perfect weight as being like placing an order for the body you want. You decide the weight that suits you, then you ask the universe to provide it. When you know you have chosen the right body and weight, you then focus on how this will look and it will come to you.

When you see others who have the body type and who are at your ideal weight, think positive thoughts about their appearance and reflect on how you would look at that same weight. Seek these people out and as you admire them and feel that emotion toward them, you are summoning the weight you desire to you. When you come across overweight people, don't let your mind dwell on their appearance. Immediately switch your thoughts back to your mind's picture of you at your perfect weight and try to feel yourself in that body.

Step 3: Receive

In order to receive what you desire, it is important that you feel happy and good within yourself. Holding on to negative thoughts about your body will prevent you from reaching your ideal. Those negative thoughts will create a powerful force and can leave you stuck in the same position you are currently. These thoughts will hold you back from changing your body. Avoid always being critical and finding in your body, as this will, in fact, attract more weight. Praise and bless every square inch of your body and focus on all the things you think are perfect about You. As you think perfect thoughts and as you feel good about You; you move to the frequency of your perfect weight and you begin truly summoning perfection.

Reward yourself with a non-food treat

Each day that you stay on track, reward yourself with a small, non-food treat. If you feel that your life lacks fulfillment, then this will start to correct that situation. Giving yourself this special, pleasurable experience in return for abiding by the rules of the diet can be an effective way to reinforce your commitment.

Things that can help generate positive emotion can include a foaming luxurious bubble bath, a nourishing face mask, an irresistible lipstick, meeting with your best friend in a tea house for a cup of green tea or going dancing with some friends at a club... This treat is as individual as you, so be creative and start to restore joy to your life - it can have remarkable results!

Don't forget to mention your treats and how you feel about them in your diet journal as well.

Body Wrap recipe for your last diet evening

The herbal body wrap recipe is just the right recipe for you on the last evening of the Cabbage Soup Diet. Body wraps are great if you want to improve, tone and tighten the look and texture of your skin. That might be especially rewarding when you notice you have experienced impressive diet weight loss.

A body wrap has both cosmetic and therapeutic benefits by reducing inches and cleansing the body of toxins. You have two options: You can reward yourself and try a special body wrap from a professional. Alternatively, you could make this simple body wrap recipe for yourself. It contains a mixture of a clay and natural sea salt that you can get in every drugstore. To supplement this simple wrap, you can add ingredients like herbs and essential oils.

Even such simple methods like adding 250 g of salt to your bath will tighten your skin and can make a big difference to your appearance.

8 ways to get rid of fattening toxins

Did you know that studies have found toxins (a synonym for poisons) - make us fat? These toxins are keeping us fat and setting us up for a number of life-threatening diseases.

Living in a toxic world

Paula Baillie-Hamilton, MD, identified that "One new chemical enters industrial use every 20 minutes, only to join many hundreds of thousands of synthetic chemicals already in use." When you consider what this means to each of us, we are surrounded by an incredible number of industrial pollutants (chemicals). The worrying thing about this is that very few of those chemicals are tested to evaluate the side-effects of exposure. "Indeed, the US has only recently begun long-term research to establish a baseline for toxins in a portion of our population. Five percent of the 1,007 women in one such study had troubling levels of polychlorinated biphenyl (or PCB 188), which has been linked to breast cancer and weight gain."

One of the best ways to help limit the impact of this relentless chemical exposure is to buy certified organic food. Food that is organic has not been treated with antibacterials, fungicides, herbicides or insecticides. "A liver overloaded with pollutants and toxins cannot efficiently burn body fat," states nutritionist Ann Louise Gittleman, PhD, CNS. "A tired, toxic liver is the number one weight-loss stumbling block."

Weight loss and a healthy, nutritious diet will help the majority of people to become healthier overall. With more healthy eating habits and adequate exercise, your body has a chance to win the battle against toxins. By cleansing your internal body with the Cabbage Soup Diet 2.0, you can help to unclog your organs and eliminate toxins - helping to give your system a chance to function better than it has for years. To help you do this even more successfully - enhance your body detoxifying in the following 8 ways:

Lower your toxic load

1) Choose foods that detoxify your body

In order to become more healthy in the future, the detoxification of the body is an important step to take. Detoxifying the body helps to restore the optimum pH and expel harmful toxins. An alkaline pH is the body's natural state - hence most detoxifying foods are primarily alkalizing.

Most vegetables and greens are alkalizing in nature, however, the list below highlights some of the most powerful detoxifying foods - the first one should come as no surprise…

Cabbage - Cabbage has gained particular popularity and fame from the Cabbage Soup Diet, which is proven to help to lose weight efficiently. Many people do not realize that they are actually receiving important detoxifying effects too.

In a review of 94 studies, it was found that a strong relationship existed between vegetables from the brassica family, such as cabbage and the reduction of cancer. The researchers doing the study found that 67% of those examined confirmed that there was a link between eating vegetables and a reduction in the likelihood of developing cancer. In addition, 70% of those studied found a clear link between cabbage consumption and a reduced risk of cancer.

In particular, lung, stomach and colon cancers are significantly reduced by eating vegetables from the brassica family. As well as having cancer-preventing phytonutrients, cabbage has high levels of vitamin C. This is also an antioxidant and aids in the protection of cells from harmful free radicals.

Garlic - This is one of the most powerful antifungal foods. Garlic has been used for thousands of years to fight off a range of different fungal infections. It is still useful today to fight things like candida yeast infections.

Beetroot - The addition of beetroot to your diet is a good option to naturally detox your liver. There is a lot of research into how this vegetable works to break up cancerous cells and the application of this as a cancer chemo (toxico) therapy. Beetroot should be eaten in moderation due to its strong properties.

Lemon - You may not have realized it, but lemon is an alkaline fruit. It is a great way to help restore a pH balance as it is one of the strongest and cheapest options available. Adding it to you diet is easy too, you can put lemon in with tea, add it to your water for some extra tang, or put it on a salad.

In actual fact, there are a great many foods that detoxify the body. Carefully choose the alternatives for your daily cabbage soup diet and afterwards. These subtle changes to your diet will ultimately contribute to your long term health.

2) Buy certified organic food

Choosing the healthier, certified organic option will reduce exposure to toxins as mentioned previously. Certain foods are more likely to have higher levels of toxins - including apples, lettuce, strawberries, spinach, peppers and green leafy vegetables. Reduce the impact of toxins by choosing organically grown food. Purchasing poultry and meat which is free of additives and chemicals is another step in the right direction and if you avoid eating the skin you'll reduce toxin exposure further still.

Chemicals can become more concentrated as they travel up the food chain. To avoid this having an impact, try cutting out carnivorous fish like sea trout. These fish eat a large number of smaller fish, taking in more of the synthetic chemicals you need to avoid.

You can replace this with fish such as cod, which is lower in the food chain and hence avoid you exposure to strongly concentrated chemicals.

3) Drink water, water, water – filtered is the best choice!

Filtered water is much better for us than the chlorinated water straight out of the tap. For starters it tastes a lot better. The charcoal and filters remove all the heavy metals, salts and chemical nasties from the water, making it much closer to water from a natural spring.

The human body is approximately seventy percent water. Within our bodies, our blood is ninety percent water and our liver, one of our most vital organs is ninety-six percent water. That's a lot of water and a major reason why you should be giving your body plenty of water to ensure good health. Since the liver is one of the major 'filter' organs of the body and it is largely water, you need to be careful that you don't expose it to toxins from your drinking water.

If you don't drink clean water you also risk any 'nasties' getting into your bloodstream and other organs - with one particular risk being the possibility of developing gall stones.

Filtering the water we drink greatly reduces the quantity of toxins present in the water and therefore reduces the toxins floating in our bloodstream and in our liver. I recommend eight glasses or more a day - which could potentially mean a lot of toxins present if you are drinking water from the tap. If you want to improve your overall health while losing weight, then get cracking and invest in a good quality filter, your body will thank you for it!

4) Avoid damaging substances

You can also keep your liver healthy by limiting the amount of alcohol, sugar, coffee (caffeine) and fats in your diet. It is also worth restricting the use of any unnecessary medications. At the same time, it helps to embrace liver boosters. Strengthen your liver with milk thistle, and consider adding soluble fiber to your diet. Fiber can be sourced from psyllium seed and pectin, and it is great for helping your body to eliminate any toxins that have accumulated.

5) Start working out regularly

As you progress with the Cabbage Soup Diet, you'll start reducing the toxic load on your system. This in turn will help your body to correctly maintain hormone levels and ensure the smooth function of the liver and the detoxification process. Increase your results by starting a regular workout and having consideration of your fitness level. Many people on the diet find they regain energy quickly, and the protein shake enhances this effect. This makes it much easier to exercise that in turn will boost your weight loss. Stick with workouts at your fitness level (and build up gradually), so that you can keep off unwanted pounds. If you continue with this routine even after you achieve your ideal weight, particularly if you exercise in the morning, then you'll raise your metabolism all day.

6) Satisfy your Vitamin B Complex demand

Cabbage is already an excellent source for vitamin B1, B2 and B6. However, the cabbage soup alone cannot cover all the essential vitamin B complex demands of your body. The Almased protein shake helps to fill the gap and provides your body with the extra vitamin Bs necessary. If you opt not to use the Almased protein shake then make sure you take a multivitamin supplement that provides you with sufficient vitamin B.

The vitamin B complexes come in many forms and each one of them has important functions in the body's natural detoxifying process. To help increase your understanding of this - I'll go through the important vitamin Bs:

Vitamin B1 (Thiamin)

This helps to fight fatigue by facilitating the release of energy from carbohydrates. It also assists in proper function of the heart, the gastrointestinal tract and the nervous system. Deficiency in Thiamin has been linked to alcoholism, schizophrenia and Alzheimer's disease. Maintaining consistently high levels of sugar, monosaturated fats (such as in junk food) and refined grains in your diet can be a leading cause of B1 deficiency.

Vitamin B2 (Riboflavin)

This helps in the metabolism and processing of food. Riboflavin also contributes to having healthy skin, hair and nails. The production of red blood cells is reliant on vitamin B2 and it activates another powerful antioxidant, Glutathione. This is important as it protects the liver against chemical toxins and it also functions as a free radical scavenger.

Vitamin B3 (Niacin)

Niacin helps the body breakdown sugars and fatty acids. The enzyme function in the nervous system is also assisted by vitamin B3 and it has been shown to provide protection against cancer. Various studies have also proved a reduction of high cholesterol levels with the correct doses of niacin.

Vitamin B6 (Pyridoxine)

An essential micronutrient and one of the vitamin B complexes, pyridoxine functions in the body's metabolism, helping to break down proteins for amino acids, as well as metabolize fats and carbohydrate. It assists a detoxification process which clears formaldehyde from the body. Cabbage is a good source of this vitamin, and one cup of cabbage provides 10% of your recommended daily Vitamin B6 intake.

Vitamin B12 (Cobalamin)

Cobalamin has a critical role to play in the human body, as the Vitamin B12 complex is found in every cell in our bodies. The presence of this vitamin in the body is a crucial factor in the maintenance of the chemical balance of the body. For dieters, it is important to understand that Vitamin B12 is needed to process fatty acids. The cobalamin complex also processes amino acids and works side by side with folic acid in the creation of normal blood cells. Cobalamin is also linked with healthy nervous tissues and fat-soluble toxic chemicals are eliminated from the body with the help of B12. This vitamin also mitigates reactions to sulfites and preservatives.

7) Herbs and Spices - Powerful and Effective in Detox

There are many herbs and spices which you can use for adding flavor to your cabbage soup. The bonus with herbs is that they have great cleansing and healing capabilities. In fact, many modern medicines exist today thanks to the development of herbal medicines in the past. Here is a small overview of some herbs and their benefits, to give you more inspiration for seasoning the soup recipes presented in the next chapter.

Parsley

This garnish - used as decoration on many dishes - is all too often left uneaten by most people. The strong flavor when eaten alone is one reason for this. However, it is this taste that represents parsley's phytochemical compound, known as polyacetylenes, which reacts strongly against cancer causing carcinogens.

Parsley also has fantastic results inhibiting the carcinogens found in tobacco smoke. This herb helps to regulate our body's production of prostaglandin and hence controls tumor growth. Parsley can add flavor to a number of dishes, so you don't have to always eat it alone if you don't particularly enjoy the taste. Consuming this herb regularly will provide many benefits which make it worth embracing it's strong flavor.

Oregano

Oregano is a herb that is popular in many Italian dishes. This herb abounds in an antioxidant known as quercitin and a phytochemical called farnesol. These two both have strong anti-cancer properties, with research demonstrating quercitin limits the growth and increase in number of breast cancer cells. In tests, the growth of mammary tumors has been seen to slow when adequate levels of quercitin are digested. The phytochemical farnesol is known for the fact that it limits skin cancer growth.

Turmeric

The turmeric spice is usually found in curries. It contains a yellow substance called curcumin, which gives curry the yellow color. This spice is great for aiding the liver's detoxification and cleansing phases. It helps to inhibit carcinogens found in charcoal grilled meats, cancer cell growth and also the development of polyps within the gastrointestinal tract. Curcumin also assists in slowing cell proliferation in prostate cancer cells.

Rosemary

Traditionally, rosemary has been added to lamb dishes, but it is also popular in soups, stews, vegetable dishes and with rice. This herb holds a phytochemical called carnasol that is a useful for detoxification.

In particular, this carnasol substance is useful for detoxifying the body of cancer causing substances. There is also evidence to indicate that this phytochemical limits development of skin cancer and lung cancer.

8) Ensure an Acid-Base pH Balance

I touched on the importance of the correct pH balance in chapter 2. When the average urine pH drops below 6.5, it shows that the body's buffering system is overwhelmed and a state of "autotoxication" exists. When this happens, it is important to lower acid levels. You can neutralize your excess acids by the intake of base substances, which containing minerals and trace elements to help excrete excess acids.

The top 7 most common mistakes

There are a great many ways that people sabotage their desire and efforts to lose weight. Understanding the things that can ruin your diet efforts is the first step to avoiding this problem.

Mistake No. 1: Assuming your choices are better than they actually are

From fruit juice to bran flakes, it's easy to believe your food choices are healthier than they actually are.

When you read a label that says 'lightly sweetened', it sounds like it will be healthy. The problem is, you need to look at many phrases such as this in context. This frequently abused claim in fact has no formal definition, so it will often be placed on cereal boxes or on fruit juice containers. In fact, many of the 'lightly sweetened' products are loaded with various sweeteners. Need proof? Look at Kellogs Smart Start. This cereal states slightly sweetened on the box, yet it actually contains more sugar per cup than a full serving of Oreo cookies! What's more - this is just one of many examples.

The solution: Go a little deeper when choosing products and take the time to read the ingredient and nutrition information - this can paint a much more accurate picture about the product. If you're buying bran flakes for your cabbage soup diet cheat, read the label carefully and buy only sugar-free bran.

Another common mistake that many people make is to eat a can of fruit and think this is more or less the same as a plateful of fresh fruits. The problem is, there is often a lot of sugar added in the preserving process or in added syrup. On top of that, much of the nutritional value can be lost during processing.

Another common mistake: Substituting fruit juices for whole fruits.

You may wonder whether fruit juice is healthier than soda - and the answer is most definitely Yes. However, juice is also a much more concentrated source of sugar than regular fruit, providing far less nutrients than you get from whole fruits. What's more - fruit juice is far less satisfying - which is important when you are on a diet. The fact is, you won't feel nearly as full after having a glass of juice as you will if you eat a piece of fruit. Instead, you take in a lot more calories and still feel hungry at the end of it.

The solution: Whole, unprocessed, fresh fruit should be the ideal choice on your fruit days. If you eat a wide variety, even if only small amounts, then you'll be on the right track to ensure you have access to a range of different nutrients. If you prefer fruit smoothies from time to time, then make them with a base of 100% fresh fruit.

If you buy pre-packaged foods, take your time and read the labels thoroughly. Don't fall into the trap of picking something that is 'masquerading' as health food. Even products in the health food section of the supermarket can trip you up - it's essential that you read the labels.

Mistake No. 2: Eating too much

Overestimating how much food you truly need is one of the most common mistakes. Many people believe that they should feel not just satisfied after a meal, but stuffed! The problem that I think arises for many people is that they then lose touch with the sensation of having had enough food.

Some people also believe that if bigger portions are suggested, then they can simply eat those large, maximum sized portions on that day of the Cabbage Soup Diet. Use your commonsense and while you are on the diet, take this opportunity to start getting familiar with your bodies signs of when you are full. It will help you to avoid overeating during the diet and also in the future.

The solution: Remain conscious of portion sizes, especially regarding the special meals on day 5, 6 and 7. The only exception is cabbage soup, which you can have as much of as you want. By having this as a starter, you'll avoid overeating at each of your meals.

Mistake No 3: Not eating enough cabbage soup

It may seem that overeating and under-eating are at opposite ends of the scale when it comes to making mistakes in your daily diet. However, many people may actually not be eating regularly enough to keep their metabolism ticking over as it should. In order to lose weight, you may try eating more regularly and eating less at each sitting.

By doing this, you'll keep your blood sugar at a steady level, preventing any insulin spikes and keeping your metabolism at its peak. This reduces fat storage and boosts metabolism - which results in decreased weight gain.

The solution: Eat the allowed food or cabbage soup every 3 - 4 hours, so you don't have those peaks and troughs of over and under-eating throughout the day.

Mistake No 4: Eating too much salt

If you're one of those people who automatically add salt to everything you eat, start weaning yourself away from this habit. Taste your food and enjoy it's natural flavor and try to be little less heavy handed with the salt when preparing your meals. Too much salt can be a major cause of heart disease in the long term - in the short term, too much salt causes you to gain water weight making you look heavier than you may truly be.

The solution: Try to cut out the salt in your diet - even if this means doing so gradually, and use a good organic, low-sodium vegetable stock when making your cabbage soup. I'll go into a bit more detail about this later on.

Mistake No. 5: Cooking only one cabbage soup recipe and becoming fed-up!

The biggest drawback of the diet for many people is the idea of eating the one thing over and over again. Believe me I sympathize with where you are coming from, which is why I have stressed variety and given hints on ways to 'shake things up' a bit. Even when you cook some cabbage soup that is great on the first sitting, by the time you've eaten it 8 or more times in a row, you'll be getting tired of eating it! Unfortunately, with the Cabbage Soup Diet
- *the soup is the key…*

That means you need to really get your cabbage soup right. To make delicious cabbage soup, make sure you begin by not overcooking the veggies. The cabbage will become 'slimy' and taste strong and sulphurous.

Throughout the diet, you'll be eating the soup a lot. Take your time to get it right so that you don't lose faith because of tasteless or disgusting soup. The biggest mistake you could make is to dump everything into a big pot with water and boil it for hours - that really will be a sulfurous, disgusting mess. (Hint - sulfur = that rotten egg smell!)

After many years of refining the cabbage soup used in the diet, I came up with the delicious recipes that I've included in chapter four of this book. You really can't imagine the difference it makes to invest some time in making your soup carefully. By taking things in steps you'll have an enjoyable soup - which is truly worthwhile, as the soup is the mainstay of the diet.

Mistake No. 6: Artificial sweeteners

In older cabbage soup diet plans there were some that allowed artificial sweeteners. I won't ban you from using them during diet week, but really don't recommend them either. Why? Well let me share a few 'home truths' about artificial sweeteners.

The problem with artificial sweetener is that it fools the body in such a way that it actually increases cravings. These chemical products don't provide any nutrition, and can actually poison your system. Here's what happens. When you drink something with an artificial sweetener your body registers that sweetness as carbohydrate. It then gets ready to process the sugar - only nothing happens.

So now your body requires the carbohydrates that it believes is coming thanks to the artificial sweeteners. The sweeteners initiate a chemical action. As there is no carbohydrate for the action to be carried out on, your body demands more carbohydrates. Nothing happens.

So your body again demands more carbohydrate. Still nothing happens. You are caught in a cycle that will not end until you succumb to the craving somehow.

So how do you satisfy the cravings? Chocolates, Cookies, Ice cream, Chips? Most of my readers who didn't finish the cabbage soup diet week reported that they used artificial sweeteners in their coffee/tea. Subsequently, the hunger and cravings they experienced while on the cabbage soup diet week did drive them crazy.

The evidence

A good indication of how this cycles has begun to creep into our lives is the evidence you can see with your own eyes. Take a look at people and their body size a generation ago. That's the generation that didn't have artificial sweeteners or diet soda - and that's the generation of people who didn't become overweight. Don't believe me? Get out some old photos and take a look for yourself.

Of course, a bunch of old photos isn't scientific evidence, but if you want to know the science behind the link between obesity and sweetener, then consider this. In a study carried out and published in the Journal of the American Medical Association (JAMA, May 14th, 2008, page 2137) it was cited that reduced calorie sweeteners can actually "help promote weight gain." The published article also identified that a high level of artificial sweeteners can "increase appetite for sweet foods" which will "promote overeating." I'm guessing that while you're trying to stick to a controlled diet - the last thing you need is an increased appetite for sweets and more overeating!

The solution: Avoid artificial sweetener wherever possible. If, like most people, you add the artificial sweetener to your obligatory coffee, then why not resist temptation altogether and drink a healthier cup of green tea instead?

Mistake No. 7 - Breaking the diet too fast

Your successful weight loss and the health benefits of this may all be lost, with harmful after effects if the diet week is not "broken" in the right way. In fact, to get the best effects, it is important you have strong nutrition management after the diet is over.

Your greatest post-diet danger lies in eating too frequently and getting back into the habit of having too much fast food at a time. After completing the diet week your body and mind will be in a sensitive condition, so try not to overload it suddenly with a large amount of unhealthy food. This could lead to acute attacks of indigestion and may produce a number of other serious side-effects. Last, but by no means least, you'll start to pile on the pounds quicker than you lost them…

I promised you that I won't expect you to 'go it alone' after the diet week, so in chapter 5 I'll give you my healthy and effective post-diet suggestions. This is just the thing you need to ensure you stay on the right track after the cabbage soup diet week.

How to reduce common side effects like headache and fatigue

The Cabbage Soup Diet 2.0 is a rapid weight loss concept. You'll be making some huge changes in your health in just a few short days. The cleansing and detoxifying process can unfortunately cause a few minor ailments in that first few days (although the longer term benefits more than outweigh this). The most common of these ailments are headache or fatigue. With the knowhow that I'm going to share however, you'll be able to significantly reduce any troublesome side effects and reap the rewards of improved health and wellbeing.

What to do when you feel light-headed

The main cause of this is when energy levels (carbohydrates) take a dive. When this happens, you need a food that can correct that sugar dip fast. Fruit is one of the best healthy options, as it will release carbohydrate into your body most rapidly. On vegetable days, having vegetables which contain high levels of sugar will help. Examples of vegetable options include carrots, beets or parsnips. I've already mentioned the benefits of nibbling carrots when you get hunger cravings, so this is an added incentive to have some of these handy while on the diet.

How a green algae can help against fatigue and faintness

Weight loss diets in general can have two unpleasant side effects - fatigue and faintness. These are both signs that your body is stressed by environmental toxins.

Chlorella pyrenoidosa is a species of fresh water green algae (e.g King Chlorella). This alga detoxifies heavy metals and pesticides from the body, while promoting the absorption of vitamins, minerals and amino acids.

Sometimes coffee makes sense

You know by now my rules regarding coffee and weight loss, so the following hint might sound a bit contradictory. As they say - rules were made to be broken… If you're experiencing headaches while dieting, then the most beneficial thing may be to drink a cup of coffee. This is because coffee will help you boost energy levels and help to correct the underlying cause of the headache.

10 bonus tips for best results

1) While dieting, eat your largest meal for the day in the middle of the day.

2) Have a light, early dinner and end each diet day with a protein shake
1 hour before bedtime.

3) Chew each bite of food thoroughly to help your body register when you are full.

4) Do not drink liquids with meals. Wait until after the meal and follow your food with a warm peppermint or ginger tea - which is great for digestion.
Get the maximum success by starting your meals with the cabbage soup.

5) Got a chocolate craving? The smell of vanilla can help stop this. Try lighting some vanilla scented candles to create a soothing atmosphere and help you get past the cravings.

6) When using olive oil for your soup or vegetables, you deserve the highest quality of extra-virgin olive oil you can get. You'll only use a little of this nutritious, healthy oil at a time - so don't scrimp too much on this product.

7) Replace vinegar with apple cider when dressing salads. This further reduces cravings and can help with melting the pounds away.

8) Excuse-proof your exercise program by planning ahead and developing strategies to help you stick to your fitness plan. Exercise with a friend to help you stay motivated.

9) Focus on getting through one day at a time - before you know it this will quickly add up!

10) Last but not least - keep going even if you slip up! Don't become negative or disheartened, instead forgive yourself, promise to do better and get straight back to following the plan.

Frequent questions from my readers

Can I switch the cabbage soup diet days around? I was a ding dong and started this diet on the week that included the 4th of July and another planned dinner with friends. Tomorrow will be day 4 for me (banana day) and was wondering if I could do day 5 tomorrow and then day 4? Since July 4th is on a meat day, I believe I will be fine. Thank you!

The reason for the food order given is to keep your insulin level balanced out and to help you avoid any cravings over the course of the week. On day four usually people have big cravings for sweets and unhealthy food. That's why bananas (or the allowed substitutions) are important at that time. They are high in carbohydrates, which help you to overcome sugar cravings. Please keep in mind that you will not get the benefit of this if you switch day 4 and 5.

Can I have a soy protein shake with unsweetened almond milk in place of milk? I don't drink milk. Almond milk has 40 calories for 8 ounces. Also, how many shakes a day are allowed?

Almond milk is a great alternative to cow or soy milk, especially for the weight conscious. Unsweetened almond milk is lower in calories, is very nutritious and contains little or no saturated fat. For the cabbage soup diet days I recommend protein shakes made with almond milk twice a day. The exception is the banana diet day. On this day I recommend a banana shake based on almond milk four times a day. If you then still want to eat "plain" bananas, this is also no problem. If you are undertaking the Cabbage Soup Diet 2.0 plan with Almased, you may choose almond milk instead of skim milk with this shake as well.

Will I really lose 10 pounds in a week?

This depends on how much weight you have to lose. If you're severely over weight or have gained weight quickly, then yes you will. If you have only a few pounds to lose, then the loss is more likely to be less. If you are only a little overweight, you will more likely see an average loss of 3-4 pounds at least; but probably more.

Another important factor determining weight loss is how many diets you have done in the past. If you've tried almost every diet going, then your weight loss might not be as impressive as it would if you were a "diet virgin".

Here is my promise to you: If you stick close to our diet, then you may achieve excellent results - even if you're already an experienced dieter. Good Luck!

Why do I seem to be gaining weight instead of losing it with the cabbage soup diet?

Everyone's body reacts different. Some people don't see any tangible weight loss until the last day of the cabbage soup diet. Others gain some weight the first days, but this turns around as their body adjusts. In the end they feel lighter and have usually dropped some pounds.

Your weight loss may also depend on how often you've been on the cabbage soup diet or another quick weight loss program in the past, as well as how overweight you are. If you repeat this diet too often, then the weight loss effect might decrease. That's why I recommend you don't do the cabbage soup diet more than 3 – 4 times per year.

Another important aspect in weight loss is whether your sodium (salt) intake per day. The more salt in your diet, the more water is retained in the body and this leads to weight (water) gain. That's why I recommend the use of low sodium bouillon cubes or low sodium salt in your soup recipes.

Here is maybe the most common reason for weight gain, although it is not yet fully understood. I discussed already how important a perfect Acid-Base Balance is for a good metabolism. If this is out of balance this could impact your weight. To check on this, test your body's acidity with pH Strips. In case you need to lower your acid level check my recommendations in chapter two.

I can't drink milk, are there any substitutes?

If you are following the Cabbage Soup Diet 2.0 with the Almased protein shake, then it should be fine to use water instead of milk. Soy milk should be used for the banana day and may be used throughout if you prefer this option to water.

Can Stevia be used to sweeten tea or cranberry juice?

Here is my opinion on Stevia as a possible sweetener. Other than Aspartam, it doesn't really affect your insulin level and that is good. Stevia won't therefore cause the strong hunger feelings that other sweeteners can.

However, there is another fact about Stevia that you should know: The FDA has refused to approve Stevia - the reason for this being its possible cancer-causing effects. My aim is not to pollute your body but to detoxify it. While it is up to you at the end of the day, I would suggest it would be a far healthier decision to omit Stevia.

Note - The reason for allowing the cranberry juice is the fact, that it is sour and hence most people are not likely to drink it in large quantities... By adding Stevia to the cranberry juice you are defeating the very purpose of putting it in to begin with.

Some cabbage soup diet plans allow artificial sweeteners, but you don't recommend them. Why?

Artificial sweeteners influence your insulin level in a negative way (as discussed in chapter 3). This can cause cravings and might make you very hungry. The aim during the diet week is to break the vicious insulin cycle of 'eating sweet – getting hungry – eating sweet – getting hungry' and so on… If you use artificial sweeteners, they could have the opposite effect and perpetuate that cycle.

Chapter 4: Cook delicious cabbage soup the fast and easy way!

My Cabbage Soup Recipe 2.0

I'd like to share my new favorite recipe with you now – I call it the cabbage soup recipe 2.0. To get the great taste and the spices just right, I invested some additional time into comparing it to other quick, basic cabbage soup recipes. It's well worth investing your time and effort into making your soup really tasty, because as I've said many times - THE SOUP IS THE KEY TO THE DIET.

Although the preparation time is a little longer than it was in the older recipe, this will actually save you time overall, as the cooking time is reduced. Here's how I make my favorite version of the soup:

Cabbage Soup Recipe 2.0

1 small head of cabbage
2 carrots
1 bunch of celery
4 tomatoes
2 red peppers
2 onions
2 leeks
1 tablespoon of olive oil
1 tablespoon of yellow curry powder
1 tablespoon of chopped caraway
2 fresh garlic cloves
1.5 l (52 oz) water
2 cubes organic vegetable stock
2 small dried chili peppers, chopped
Lemon grass, fresh parsley

Directions:

1. Wash and chop the vegetables. Lightly sauté the onion and garlic with the olive oil in a large stockpot. Stir in the caraway. Cook for a few minutes.

2. Add the slower cooking vegetables such as the red pepper, leeks, carrots, celery and so on, along with the cubes of organic stock (use low sodium) and the water. If you would like a sweeter-tasting soup, then add extra carrots!

3. Bring the soup to a boil and add the faster-cooking veggies and herbs (tomatoes, parsley, chili, curry and lemon grass).

4. Add your finely shredded cabbage LAST, and only cook the soup until the cabbage turns bright green. This should usually take about 10 minutes of simmering - and you're done!

Take the soup off the heat. You can then eat it as it is, or put your delicious soup into storage containers to see you through the first few days of your diet.

The Prototype Cabbage Soup Recipe

If you prefer the spartan approach, then you'll love the classic cabbage soup recipe for its ease and simplicity.

Here's how you make the soup:

1 head of cabbage
6 large onions
2 green peppers
1-2 cans of diced tomatoes
1 bunch of celery
1 package of Lipton Onion Soup Mix
1-2 cubes of vegetable broth (low sodium)

Directions:
1) Cut the vegetables into small pieces and cover with water.
2) Bring to the boil and cook at a fast boil for 10 minutes.
Reduce the soup to a simmer and continue cooking until the vegetables become tender.

Note: This is the old 'classic' cabbage soup recipe. I find that making this version is the easiest and quickest way of preparing cabbage soup. The key to making tasty soup with this recipe is to cook your soup for only 10 minutes. Originally, it was recommended that you simmer the soup for almost an hour. From a nutritional standpoint, this simply makes no sense nowadays.

By cooking the soup for so long, you'll just end up losing the most important vitamins and minerals from the vegetables, plus you'll have tasteless, sulfurous soup.

Delicious Cabbage Soup Recipe Variations

They say 'variety is the spice of life' and when you are creative and use ingenious ideas to vary your cabbage soup, you'll be amazed how much more enjoyment and satisfaction you'll get from it. There are many different combinations and particular ingredients that will make a big difference to your soup. Options you may like to try can include crushed garlic, cumin, curry powder, caraway, basil, rosemary, sage, thyme, dill, chives, parsley, sliced mushrooms, cinnamon, cloves, nutmeg and many, many more...

On the next page I've put together some fabulous variations for your cabbage soup diet recipe. These are all great for giving your prototype cabbage soup recipe a truly delicious zing!

To use these variations, simply add the ingredients to the soup as it cooks. If you prefer a milder flavor, then try adding smaller amounts to flavor one bowl of soup.

Cabbage Soup "Munich"
1/2 cup of apple cider vinegar
1-2 teaspoon of whole caraway seeds
3 sprigs of fresh thyme (crushed) or
2 teaspoon dried thyme

Cabbage Soup "Florence"
3 cloves of garlic (crushed)
3/4 cup of chopped Italian parsley (flat leaf)
4 fresh oregano leaves (crushed)

or 1 teaspoon of dried oregano
some basil

Cabbage Soup "Bombay"
3 cucumbers, peeled and sliced
2 teaspoon ground turmeric
2 teaspoon ground cumin
some saffron, if at hand

Cabbage Soup "Buena Vista"
2 jalapeño peppers, finely chopped
4 teaspoon chili powder

Cabbage Soup "Honolulu"
1-2 teaspoon ginger
1 teaspoon hot sauce

Cabbage Soup "South Western"
chopped cilantro
1/2 teaspoon chili powder
some cumin

Cabbage Soup "Casablanca"
1/2 teaspoon curry powder mixed into the cooking soup
chopped fresh mint leaves for garnish on top when serving

Cabbage Soup "Peking"

Shrimp or fish bouillon
1 tablespoon soy sauce
some fresh bean sprouts

Cabbage Soup "Chanterelle"

Chanterelle mushrooms
a pinch of thyme and rosemary
with tomatoes for a wonderful French taste
without tomatoes for an exotic oriental sensation

A dash of seasoning

When preparing the cabbage soup recipe, don't be afraid to adjust seasonings to suit your own tastes. To help keep the soup healthy, aim to omit flavorings or ingredients with high-sodium levels. Instead opt for bouillon cubes, soup mixes or low-sodium or salt-free versions.

My tip: Try Mrs. Dash® Salt-Free Seasoning Blends.

These add delicious taste not only to your soup, but can be used when cooking a broad range of things, from soups to salads to seafood.

The best thing that I've found about this product is that it's all-natural and the all-purpose blend of 14 different herbs and spices is the perfect way to bring out the unique flavor of any dish. The Mrs. Dash® Original Blend includes onion, black pepper, parsley, basil, orange peel and tomato, which can really spice up and enhance the flavor of any dish. There are also other combinations available, so pick one that is appealing for you: www.successful-diet-cabbage-soup.com/resource-center.html

Reduce flatulence, aches and pains

Different people will react in different ways when they change their diet. Various foods can cause a range of physical responses. Some people can seem to eat anything and they have no side effects, others can get gas from the most bland of foods. If you discover you have any problems when you first change your diet, then the following list of useful, natural remedies could be just what you need.

Cumin
Cumin is a good option if you're looking for a spice that will relieve flatulence. This is a great choice for flavoring your soup and if you enjoy the flavor, make sure to try the 'Bombay' cabbage soup recipe. If you find the taste is a little too strong for your liking, then don't worry. There are other herbs and spices that have similar properties, including peppermint, sage, dill, fennel and thyme.

Chamomile Flowers
Chamomile flowers can be added to your soup, or even to a tea if you

like. This flower has quite a neutral taste, so it provides a number of benefits without creating an overwhelming flavor.

Ginger

Ginger is a versatile choice, making a good drink when mixed with lemon juice, as well as being giving added flavor in your soup or to a vegetable plate or stir-fry. It is most useful for soothing the intestinal tract, relieving flatulence and helping digestion in general.

If you want to have a wide range of herbs and try out different flavors while still getting the health benefits, then you should look for those from the carrot and mint families. This includes herbs such as basil, coriander, garlic, marjoram, rosemary, oregano, lavender and nutmeg.

Eat slowly!

In order to shut off your body's gasworks, start by eating more slowly. I mentioned the benefits of this in chapter three, as eating slowly has a more satiating effect. Take the time to relax over your meal and chew your food thoroughly. Wolfing down food will mean it can enter the intestine before it is fully digested.

There are a number of other ways to avoid problems with gas - and this includes the following: Smoking, drinking carbonated drinks, chewing gum and gulping water at drinking fountains.

Save 80% of your preparation and cooking time - and save money!

When corporate entities promote health fads, they are often far more worried about their bottom line than yours! The truth is, they often want to make a big profit and will sell all number of pills, gadgets, potions, fitness equipment and gym memberships in a bid to part you from your money! The Cabbage Soup Diet is NOT like that. The diet is not about making a profit from you by playing on your emotions about losing weight. In actual fact, you could make the change to the Cabbage Soup Diet for just a couple of dollars a day!

With the Cabbage Soup Diet 2.0, the only measurements you have to make are of the ingredients you put into your nutritious meals. There is no counting of calories, no adding and subtracting of grams of fat and no complicated math involved in working it all out.

If you're really on a tight budget, you could still achieve good results by replacing the Almased with low fat milk (although with Almased the diet is easier). It truly is about your health and weight loss, not about parting you from a mountain of your money…

The following are my most highly recommended ideas for saving even more time and money when you are following the Cabbage Soup Diet 2.0.

1) The perfect cooking method

Overboiling any vegetable will cause it to lose much of its nutritional value. When cooking your soup, simply bring it to a boil and then simmer for 10 minutes. You know it's ready when the cabbage turns bright green.

By cooking for a shorter amount of time, the preparation of your soup is not only completed more quickly, you know the vitamins and nutritional value of the soup remains high.

2) The right cooking gear

These days, there are a wide range of time saving devices and gadgets that help you to save loads of precious time in the kitchen. That makes preparing nutritious meals easier and less time consuming. Here are some essential items for helping you to speed up your cooking time and make it more pleasant:

- A large stockpot for your cabbage soup
- A coated pan for steaming vegetables the low fat way - if you have one, a wok is even better…
- A steamer to help with quick and healthy vegetable preparation
- A blender to mix smoothies, your cabbage soup or to whip up a salad dressing
- Several cutting boards, to save you time on cleaning between chopping meat and chopping veggies)

- A microwave oven to heat up your soup - you'll find this indispensable!
- Tupperware containers for freezing and storing your cabbage soup

When you have great tools to work with, you'll find that cooking becomes simpler, speedier and a lot more fun! Once you've got the cooking done, the next section covers more time saving tips.

Freezing Your Cabbage Soup

When you're short on time during the week, then it can help to plan ahead and set aside a little time on the weekend to make some cabbage soup in advance. The soup is perfect for freezing, so you simply work out what you need for the diet and prepare and freeze the number of servings you think you'll need. Freezing the Cabbage Soup makes it super easy to stick with eating delicious diet meals at a later date.

The Cabbage Soup recipe is one of the best types of soups for reheating. When you prepare and freeze fresh and nutritious foods having cooked the soup, this is the perfect way to ensure you stick with your diet and have highly nutritious food as well. To manage this successfully, you simply need some containers for freezing and a little time to prepare the soup ready for your freezer.

Here are the steps to take once you've prepared the soup and are ready to freeze it:

Step 1: Let the soup cool

Begin by setting your soup aside for an hour or two until it reaches room temperature. Putting hot soup in the freezer could result in freezer burn, or the lid can pop as steam collects. When it is so simple to avoid, it is commonsense to just allow the soup to cool first.

Step 2: Put your soup into Tupperware bowls

I like to put my soup into Tupperware bowls, as it is one of the easiest ways to divide the soup into the amount you are likely to eat each day. It is never wise to defrost and refreeze foods, even the cabbage soup.

If you don't have bowls, any storage container is fine, simply ladle out the soup to ensure you have sensible size portions and don't let any go to waste!

Step 3: Fold a paper towel and place over the soup in the Tupperware container

A piece of folded paper towel placed over the soup before the lid goes on and it goes into the freezer is a good way to protect from freezer burn.

Step 4: Seal the soup carefully before putting it in the freezer

Finally, make sure that all the containers are carefully sealed before placing in the freezer. Soup prepared in advance will need to be thawed out, so you will need to remember this when it comes time to using it. I prefer to reheat mine in the microwave to save time once it has defrosted, however you could heat it on the stovetop if you so desire (don't cook, just heat). I also like to add some of my favorite herbs before heating for a bit of added zing.

When you take the time to carry out a little advanced preparation it can be a big time saver.

Note: Use your soup within two months of freezing. Make sure you always use a clean ladle, chopping board, containers and utensils to avoid contamination. Do not thaw and refreeze the soup, this will not only compromise the flavor, but also the safety of your soup.

Frequent questions from my readers

Cheats I have seen - Are cheats really OK and are there any others? I've seen versions of the diet that allow you to add 1 tablespoon of low-fat sour cream and up to 2 teaspoons of shredded low fat mozzarella cheese to flavor the soup and add texture. Are these cheats really ok or not? Also, are there any others I can use? This is my second time trying the diet and I find using these two cheats makes the soup more tolerable.

Using limited cheats is ok with the soup, but these are per day and NOT per soup portion. You may add the following:

1 tablespoon of low-fat sour cream

OR up to 2 teaspoons of shredded, low-fat mozzarella cheese
OR up to 2 teaspoons grinded cheese
OR up to 1 tablespoon olive oil

Only try one at a time, not all of them together - stick with one per day and decide which you like the best. It is possible to spread the use of the olive oil throughout the day.

For example, use some to fry your vegetables and use some to pour in the broth with the other ingredients I've listed in my Cabbage Soup Recipe 2.0.

A good olive oil will add a really great flavor to the soup. If you want to use some olive oil for your salad dressing, then remember to also deduct this quantity. Using a few cheats generally won't harm your weight loss success.
If they help you stay motivated and focused on your goal, then they are doing quite the opposite. I always think that if a few "healthy" cheats keep you away from the "bad" cheats like chocolate and cakes, then they can't be so bad as long as you only use them when absolutely necessary.

If they help you to enjoy more of the cabbage soup recipes, then you'll be more eager to eat the soup as a filler before meals even when you complete the cabbage soup diet week.

Can I use PAM Spray/no-calorie spray butter?

PAM is a non-stick cooking spray that comes in different flavors (like olive oil or butter flavor). You may use a little PAM spray, however, I don't recommend it if you are serious about detoxifying your body as well as losing weight. There are some who would argue that PAM spray, which is based on canola oil, is "the aspartame of cooking oils".

It is proven that canola oil has some undesirable health effects when it is the main source of dietary fat. For this reason, I would recommend wherever possible to stick with healthier oils, such as extra virgin olive oil. It is a more healthy way to get your dietary fat each day while following the Cabbage Soup Diet 2.

Chapter 5: How to avoid bad old habits after the Cabbage Soup Diet

The No.1 maintenance tip after the cabbage soup diet 2.0

For many people, getting the weight off is only half the battle. Once you have succeeded in getting your weight down, there is the day to day struggle to keep it down. The biggest trap you can fall into is bingeing and regaining the weight. The biggest advantage of the Cabbage Soup Diet 2.0 week is that it not only helps you lose weight, but gives you an opportunity to break free from a lifetime rollercoaster of dieting.

The diet gives your body a start on the right track, preparing you for a more healthy and nutritious diet and lifestyle. After the week of fruits, vegetables and cabbage soup, your body starts to understand how good nutritious food is again. This is the beginning of a permanent shift in your feelings about food and your attitude towards how you treat your body. After finishing the Cabbage Soup Diet you have experienced how great it feels to have a leaner body and to be better nourished.

So here it comes - my No.1-maintenance tip… Stick to the soup! Yes, you read that right. It really is that simple!

If you developed a preference for one type of soup during the diet week, then use that recipe often and have the soup as a starter before your meals. By doing this, you'll feel much better and it will help you to avoid over-eating the 'bad' stuff that will pack the pounds back on!

The great thing about this is that you don't only have to have cabbage soup to feel full. Once you've finished the diet week, you can 'mix

things up' and inject some variety with broth-based vegetable soups –
in fact, you can even get the same effect from chicken soup! Adding a
soup as a first course and then eating less for the rest of the meal is
easy to do and it is a small step that can truly help you maintain your
weight or even lose some more pounds in the long run. I've
experienced this firsthand and thousands of my readers have found
they have similar results. If you are worried that all seems a little too
easy, then I'd like to share the scientific research that backs this up:

Nutrition researcher Barbara Rolls conducted studies in the late 1990s
which demonstrate people tend to eat the same amount of food day
after day, pretty much no matter what. The Volumetrics Diet is based
in part on this very research. If you tend to eat the same amount and
you're filling up on hamburgers, pizzas or candy bars, then what if
you cut some of that out by replacing some of that volume of food
with soup? I'm sure you see where I'm going here, but here's some
more proof.

The Dramatic Satiety Difference between Soup and Water

The difference in satiety between water consumed on and as an
ingredient in soup is truly remarkable. In a study of the different
effects, one group of women was given a 270-calorie first course
before lunch. Some days that first course would be a chicken and rice
casserole. On others days they got the same casserole plus a 10 oz
glass of water. On the remaining days they got the casserole, with an
extra 10 oz of water cooked into it to make a soup.

The extraordinary result of this was that the soup reduced the calories
they ate at the lunch that followed. Not only did the women consume
about 100 calories less at lunch after the soup, they didn't feel
hungrier later. The women also found that they didn't desire an extra
helping at dinner to make up the difference. In Paris, researches
recently reported the same thing. When water was served as a
beverage with a meal it didn't enhance satiety. When the same amount
was taken as part of a soup it did. Their research also found that
chunky soup, was more satiating than strained soup.

Regularly eating soup helps you lose weight because it changes your eating patterns

In fact, research about soup's remarkable weight loss benefits has been around for a while. In 1979, Dr. Henry Jordan, a behavioral weight-control specialist, had 500 volunteers eat soup for lunch every day for 10 weeks. The result? The soup eaters consumed fewer calories when this was a regular part of their diet; with volunteers losing an average of 20% of their excess body weight. So why is this so?

The reason behind this is that soup is relatively complicated to eat. You need time and motor skills to consume it, which often causes people to eat less. Soup necessitates you sit in order to eat comfortably, plus you need a spoon and you are physically limited in the amount you can consume in each spoonful. It's not easy to gulp it down and when you put it in a larger bowl, you often 'trick' your body into believing you've had a larger portion.

Added to the physical constraints of eating soup is the various different textures, shapes and flavors to be considered. You are likely to take your time more eating it, which is another beneficial thing.

The Bottom Line: Add a tasty, low-calorie soup to your daily routine (lunch is a great choice, but you could benefit even more if you add it to dinner as well) and you will lose weight. You'll just ensure your body has less calories to burn.

Many dieters will skip this important maintenance tip, but the fact is, it is super easy to do, not to mention super effective! It may be that it just seems to simple when we have so much competing information 'sold' to us by corporate weight loss organizations. Let's face it, the weight loss industry has no interest in letting you know it could be that simple.

If you have had a weight problem, then it really is essential you find simple ways to develop a better, more nutritious diet that help you keep your weight down after dieting. Many people who think in terms of being "on" or "off" a diet fall into the trap of overeating on those "off" diet days. Avoid this by looking at the Cabbage Soup Diet 2.0 as being your chance to change your lifestyle and stick with an easy, healthy way of eating in the future. Don't make this too restrictive, as a few moderate splurges now and then can help to avoid those big binges that can really cause trouble.

So, soup on!

The most important ingredient after the cabbage soup diet

Nutrition plays a vital role in controlling your appetite and hunger, keeping these stable by providing you with essential vitamins and minerals. It ensures that your body metabolizes sugar and fat at a steady rate, as well as maintaining blood glucose levels, the burning of calories and more. A careful balance is needed to ensure that the minerals work with each other, which means it is hard to single out one particular mineral as being "the best" for weight loss. However, there is one mineral that really is worth a special mention - and that is calcium.

If your nutrition already includes sufficient levels of calcium, then congratulations! If you have experienced problems with weight loss, then you are more likely however, to have a deficiency of calcium.

Calcium: it's not just bones anymore!

Most of us understand that calcium's plays a vital role in building strong, healthy teeth and bones. However, current research is now showing that as calcium intake goes up, both body weight and body fat goes down.

A study published in an issue of the *British Journal of Nutrition* last year, identified that boosting calcium consumption increases weight loss in those whose diets are calcium deficient. Studies carried out recently have demonstrated a positive relationship between calcium intake and weight loss. Controlled weight loss studies indicate that by increasing calcium intake by the equivalent of two dairy servings per day, the chances of being overweight are likely reduced by as much as 70 percent!

Angelo Tremblay and his team at Université Laval's Faculty of Medicine discovered this during a 15-week weight loss program studying obese women. Participants consumed less than 600 mg of calcium per day on average - while the recommended daily intake is at least 1000 mg. Alongside a low calorie diet, each participant was instructed to take two tablets a day containing either a total 1200 mg of calcium or a placebo. Those who took the calcium tablets lost nearly 6 kg during the study, while the researchers found the women in the control lost only 1 kg.

"Our hypothesis is that the brain can detect the lack of calcium and seeks to compensate by spurring food intake, which obviously works against the goals of any weight loss program," explains Angelo Tremblay, holder of the Canada Research Chair in Environment and Energy Balance. "Sufficient calcium intake seems to stifle the desire to eat more."

When the necessary levels of calcium are consumed, it becomes an important part of the success of any weight loss program. Having had the opportunity to carry out research into calcium consumption, the researcher identified that more than 50% of obese women who attended the clinic run by his research team didn't consume the recommended daily calcium intake.

Professor Tremblay and his research team spent several years closely studying the links between calcium and obesity. Their initial findings were published in 2003. These studies revealed that women whose diets were low in calcium had more body fat, larger waistlines, as well as higher levels of bad cholesterol. Many of these signs were absent in women who consumed moderate to large amounts of calcium as a part of their regular diet.

A subsequent second study tracking results across a six year period revealed that the less dairy people ate, the higher their weight, levels of body fat and the larger their waistlines became. In 2007, Angelo

Tremblay and his team identified a direct link between calcium and a lower cardiovascular risk profile among dieters.

Here's how you can reach the recommended daily intake of 1000 mg of calcium per day in a natural way:

1 cup of skim milk (220 ml) =	**278 mg Calcium**
Firm cheese like cheddar or gouda (50 g) =	**350 mg Calcium**
1 cup low-fat yoghurt plain (175 g) =	**292 mg Calcium**

My Tip: Drink just one Almased Protein Shake with milk, once a day and you'll get **over 75% of the necessary calcium intake:**

1 cup of skim milk (220 ml)	**278 mg Calcium**
1 portion of Almased (35 g/3 heaped tbsp.)	**506 mg Calcium**

You can also boost your dietary calcium by eating plenty of green leafy vegetables. High levels of calcium can be found in broccoli, chicory, kale, lettuce, romaine or spinach. You'll soon discover that taking in 1000 mg of calcium every day is a breeze! When choosing dairy products that will increase your calcium levels, remember that low-calorie, fat-free milk has the same quantity of calcium as full-fat milk. This is equally so for low-fat yogurt and reduced-fat cheese.

The single biggest mistake after finishing the Cabbage Soup Diet

There are a lot of dieters who find that reaching the end of the diet is such a motivator they want to do it all again! If you've experienced great results, then this is understandable, but I urge you not to do this.

While you may feel energized after the first week, continuing on to a second week is likely to start doing your body harm. The Cabbage Soup Diet 2.0 will help you achieve great results, but it does so via a short term, highly restricted diet. The goal of this is to help give you a confidence boost, help you drop some weight and help you to detoxify ready to start a longer term, healthy and nutritious diet.

The Cabbage Soup Diet is not designed to be used as an ongoing program for sustained weight loss beyond one week.

Instead, I hope that you'll take the knowledge you've gained about nutrition and good health, using this as a launching point for a new healthier way of eating in the future.

One of the best strategies to take away from the diet is to continue eating the cabbage soup or another broth-based soup as a starter before all your meals. This helps ensure adequate nutrition and gets you to develop good, long-term eating-habits. I recommend that you wait at least several months before repeating the diet week. By waiting, you will give yourself the means to finally break free from the yo-yo dieting cycle.

My Top 5 motivation techniques for enhancing & maintaining a "thin you"

For many people the primary motivation in losing weight is to feel better about how they look. Achieving good health should, however, be the most important goal of all. The great thing about the Cabbage Soup Diet is that both of these things can be achieved at the same time.

I understand my readers desire to stick with the diet for longer after achieving good results in the first week. I cannot stress enough however, that this is not a wise idea. The great results you achieve in the first week are because the Cabbage Soup Diet gives your body a positive 'kick-start' to help you begin shedding the pounds. Long term weight loss requires a strong commitment and a slow and steady approach. I know that this can be tough, and many people have asked me how can they stay motivated when things are happening at the proverbial snail's pace?

1) Choose a weight maintenance strategy that you think works for you, then stick with that strategy after completing the diet week. If you choose soup as a starter for your strategy, then stick with that and don't lose sight of your goal.

2) When you decided to begin the Cabbage Soup Diet, you made a firm decision that you were going to take control of your weight and fitness. I have found that it is helpful to think of the excess fat as a villain stopping you from achieving your ideal weight. When you have this imagery in your mind, it will empower you to begin fighting off that fat and regaining control.

3) One way to build upon the villain idea is to think of the fatty, sugary or starchy foods as the weapons that the 'fat villain' uses against you.

When you stay away from these, you are taking control of the power. If you develop strong cravings, start working on taking control of these and not being swept along by them. One good option is not to keep those foods that trigger cravings in your home. If you do get tempted, it can be a lot more hassle to go to the store than it is to go to the fridge. Having a lot of healthy snacks that are easy to have instead will guarantee that you can stay in control and conquer those cravings!

4) Consistency is the key to achieving lasting results. In order to get there, start developing a strong, focused mindset. Find ways to manage different situations. If you are going out for dinner, for example, then have a large salad or some soup at home before going out. That way you'll avoid overdoing it during the evening and be able to enjoy yourself without any guilt about what you've eaten.

5) A dull and repetitive exercise routine can help you to lose motivation. To make sure you stick with your program, add some variety and find different ways to exercise that will keep you interested. Try jogging, swimming or cycling - or add some other physical activity that you enjoy such as a salsa or belly dance class. By doing things you enjoy, the exercise will not become a 'chore' and you'll stay on track to lose weight and improve your fitness.

Here's one of my own special tips: Try trampolining everyday. I love getting out there and jumping up and down just like a kid - but more than that - trampolining is the second quickest way to burn calories! If you spend 20 minutes jumping, it's equivalent to 30 minutes of jogging and its lots of fun! Trampoline training is even used by astronauts who are in training for space travel. I think that the rush of endorphins from the exercise is equaled by the joy that I get out of this activity - and why shouldn't you enjoy an exercise that also makes you happy.

If you slip up and find there are times when you're not keeping up with your routine, then don't get dragged down by negative thoughts. Just get back on track and stay focused on the bigger picture. Before you know it you'll be back in the swing of things and back on track to achieve the results you desire.

Simple, healthy ways to improve your diet

1) Swap fatty, oily foods for healthy choices.

When you finish the diet week, start using the changes and make conscious decisions about eating foods that will keep you fit, healthy and lean. Improving your diet is about taking out the fatty, greasy foods and maintaining your weight and health with leaner choices. Fast food and fried food are two of the biggest downfalls for many of us, so start switching these for healthier alternatives. Remember, as a general guideline, to lose weight you need only 20-60 g of fat per day; for maintaining a steady weight, you need around 60 – 80 g each day.

Here are some hints to manage this:

Eat lean meats:

Processed meats are often high in fat. To avoid this, try eating skinless chicken and fish, instead of sausages or hamburgers. If you love the taste of fried chicken, you could cut out a lot of fat by baking it instead of deep frying. Veggie burgers or a low-fat turkey sandwich are a good alternative to fatty hamburgers. Another good 'fast-food' is home- made pizza. You can buy the crust at a store and simply add your own pizza sauce and veggies. That way you can use low fat cheese and olive oil or simply leave the cheese off to ensure a tasty, healthy pizza option.

Make gradual changes:

The diet week is a great starting off point to begin to make changes. You don't have to make every change overnight. I would suggest trying a 30 day challenge or similar after completing the initial week. You can use that time to introduce a whole range of changes to ensure you develop healthier, sustainable eating habits that will keep your weight down for the long haul.

Some extra fat fighting hints:

When cooking, replace 30 g (1 oz) of unsweetened baking chocolate with 3 tablespoons of cocoa powder and 2 teaspoons of vegetable oil. Try using cottage cheese in place of cream cheese - it could save you up to 72 g of fat per cup!

Swap the whole milk for skim milk (1%).

Try replacing one whole egg with the yolk for 2 egg whites or a quarter cup of egg substitute.

**2) Take steps to replace sugary foods
with healthier sweet treats**

Sugary foods are the next important area to work on when you have started to cut out the fatty foods from your diet. Work on doing this step by step. Change sugary snacks for healthier, low carb alternatives by starting one at a time. The changes you have made to eat more low fat, low sugar foods, along with the introduction of an ongoing exercise routine will see you continue to lose weight steadily after you complete the diet week.

Some ways to make positive changes:

- **Challenge yourself**: One option to help you succeed is to have a 30 day challenge with sweet food just as you did with fatty foods. If you can go a whole month without sweets - you're on the path to success! If you don't' think you could manage that, then a gradual cutting down of sweets over that time is still a good start.

- **Have a set cheat day**: I would recommend you select one day of the week that you allow yourself to have a small number of sweets. I make my day Saturday and on that day I eat a dessert. I find that when I set aside one day, it makes it simpler to stick to not having any sweets on any other days. I also find I eat less than I used to.

- **Sweet alternatives**: Make a list of alternatives to the sweets you had in the past and then stock up on these. If you find you are craving something sweet, having these at that time will help to overcome this successfully. I think it is best to get rid of sweets from your house as well, so that you don't have that as an added temptation.

- **Drinks**: Soda or juice is high in calories. Swap this for water or fruit teas, so that you can cut those calories.

- **Whole grains**: These are a good way of reducing your carbohydrate load, so that you feel full for longer and you don't become tempted to over eat when your blood sugar drops after eating a lot of refined foods.

A few more low-carb hints:

You can reduce your calorie intake and keep your blood sugar better balanced by avoiding cola, lemonade, fruit juices and beer. These drinks have a high Glycemic Index (GI) and a high Glycemic Load (GL), which is likely to increase your levels of insulin (the fat hormone).

Swap the high GI drinks for water, fruit and herbal teas, or sugar free fruit and vegetable juices (mix these with 2/3 water).

Remember to eat high fiber food. Chew your food and eat at a relaxed pace. This helps your body to have time to register when you are full, which will mean you can maintain your weight more successfully, as you will avoid over eating. High fiber food will help to keep you full for longer and maintain a stable level of insulin.

If you have fatty foods or meals with a high GI, then try to avoid pairing multiple foods like this. Examples of the kinds of combinations to avoid include white bread with both butter and jam or cheese, pizza with cheesy garlic bread, croissants with chocolate, roast pork with French fries and so on.

If you enjoy a glass of wine with your meal (it is a good source of anti-oxidants!), try to select dry wines.

Sugar can be used to add taste to food, but I like to think of it as a source of flavor, not nutrition!

10 great ideas for preparing healthy low fat or low carbohydrate snacks

- A handful of dry apricots, mangos or paw paws (papayas). These tasty, dried fruits are an excellent alternative to sweets with processed sugar or as an after lunch "dessert". As an added bonus, they are rich in vitamins and 100% fat free.
- Kefir strawberry mix: Combine 1 cup kefir (3.5%) with 120 g (4.2 oz) of strawberries in a high pot. Flavor the mixture with 1 teaspoon of honey.
- Blueberry mix: Blend 1 cup of low fat milk, 120 g (4.2 oz) of blueberries and 1 small bowl of frozen yoghurt.
- 300 g sweet cherries (10.5 oz), washed. Delicious without anything added!
- Have a low fat fruit or soy bar
- Have 15 g (0.5 oz) of mozzarella with 3 sliced radishes. Season them with pepper and freshly chopped parsley
- Prepare 2 fresh figs with an Italian bread stick
- Slice 220 g (7.7 oz) of honeydew melon with 20 g (0.75 oz) of Parma ham
- Have crisp bread with 3 thin slices of lean roast beef and add 1/4 of a cucumber, sliced
- Prepare 2 tomatoes with 1/2 a cup of cottage cheese

Chapter 6: The essentials of keeping the new you - long after you've finished the Cabbage Soup Diet 2.0!

Diet traps to avoid in every situation

During the week spent following the Cabbage Soup Diet 2.0, you'll go without any junk food - filling your body with healthy and nutritious food throughout that time. Following on from this, your body will be ready for a new way of eating and future good nutrition.

In chapter 3 I told you how regularly eating a lot of junk food is one of the biggest mistakes you can make. High calorie food that holds little nutrition, such as pizzas, burgers, fish and chips, sweets and crisps are at the top of the list of things to avoid - and I'll talk about this more in the next section.

Your body and your mind will be altered after the week spent on the diet. In this period, you need to make sure you don't go over the top and take in too much junk food after you have cleansed these foods from your system. If you do overdo it, you may find you experience indigestion. It is also possible to pack on the weight more quickly if you do this after the diet week.

The changes will stay with you as you adjust your eating habits not only following the diet week, but also in the future as you start to adopt a healthier outlook and better eating habits. Including soup as a starter following the diet and avoiding junk food is the key to eating more healthily in the future. Don't fall into the trap of adjusting your diet and eating healthily for only a few weeks then starting up your old habits again.

Handling your cravings sensibly is the key to staying healthy in the long run and not finding yourself back where you started before beginning the diet.

Here's why cravings are so hard to handle:

Junk food is addictive!

In Australia, scientists discovered that junk food is addictive and this is why people can find it so difficult to break free from eating this food regularly. Understanding that too much junk food can lead to health problems, researchers presented their research at a meeting in Adelaide held by The Australian Society for Medical Research.

Throughout the 2 months of research conducted, the scientists fed laboratory rats food that was rich in sugar and fat. The goal was to cause them to gain weight and become 'anxious' when food was replaced.

Zhi Yi Ong, a post-graduate student from the University of South Australia, found that there were rats that would chose to go hungry instead of eating healthy food. Ms. Ong stated that ,*"It seems like the desire for junk food has overridden their hunger signals, they would rather eat nothing ... than consume the chow as their energy source".*

The researchers studied two groups of rats. One group was fed different biscuits, hazelnut spread, peanut butter, sugar-loaded cereals and cheese and bacon-flavored snacks. The other group of rats was only fed healthy food pellets. Over a 3-day period the scientists then monitored the rats and found that the rats fed junk food were more agitated and spent time running around far more than the 'healthy' group.

Ms. Ong said that, "When not with the junk food they became more anxious ... they were probably suffering from junk food withdrawal".

You need to consume more and more junk food in order to have the same feeling

During the first stage of the study, the scientists were focused on the behavior of the rats. In the second phase, research scientists tested to determine the levels of dopamine being processed in the brains of the rats. *"We're speculating junk food can down-regulate (desensitize) the reward pathway in our brains. So if you have consumed too much, you have to consume more and more in order to feel the same happy feeling,"* says the researcher.

You're not over the hump yet!

What exactly does this research mean for you? Well, it is clear that following the Cabbage Soup Diet 2.0 is a highly effective way to rid yourself of the 'addiction' to junk food. What is important, however, is to understand you can't let yourself fall back into the old habits. Don't let junk food creep back into your diet after getting through the diet week.

Be firm with yourself once you have got through the diet week. Don't forget that if you were a junk food addict, then you can still return to that after completing the Cabbage Soup Diet. Following the diet for 1 week will not be enough to be rid of this. If you've been remaining healthy and avoiding unprocessed foods for some weeks now, then you are still likely to find there are days when the desire for junk food can be overwhelming.

Humans can react just the same way to junk food as the rats in the nutrition studies carried out in Australia.

Once you get hooked on junk food, then you'll end up wanting to eat only that - even to the point where you would rather go hungry than eat healthy food. It will reach a point where you will no longer find the taste of nutritious fruit and vegetables satisfying. The preference you have for junk food can develop really quickly. The more often you eat this food, the greater your cravings will be and the larger the quantities you will desire to satisfy the cravings.

Don't try using the Cabbage Soup Diet 2.0 to begin yo-yo dieting. There are some who think that if they have one week of junk food, one of cabbage soup and so on - then they can avoid the need to adopt more healthy eating habits as a long term solution for good health. As I've mentioned, repeating the Cabbage Soup Diet week too often will mean that it will not be as effective as it would be otherwise. You'll end up piling on the pounds instead of losing them.

Some goldmines for fast food junkies

To help you overcome those cravings for junk food - here are some of my 'easy swap' strategies for avoiding the junk food urge.

Easy Swap # 1: Carob or very dark chocolate (70% cacao), instead of a creamy chocolate bar. You can have these snacks 3 days a week - Lose around 12 - 15 pounds in a year.

Easy Swap # 2: Have coffee with skim milk instead of "coffee house" latte.
You can have this 5 days a week - Lose 18 - 20 pounds in a year.

Easy Swap # 3: Have whole grain cereal with skim milk instead of a bran muffin. You can have this 3 times a week - Lose 14 - 15 pounds in a year.

Easy Swap # 4: Have mustard instead of mayonnaise on sandwiches. You can have this 3 times a week - Lose 12 - 13 pounds in a year.

Easy Swap # 5: Have a turkey sandwich with lettuce and tomato instead of a cheeseburger and fries. You can have this 3 times a week - Lose 8 - 10 pounds in a year.

Easy Swap # 6: Have 180 g (6.3 oz) baked potato with sour cream instead of 150 g (5.3 oz) of french fries. You can have this 3 times a week - Lose 10 pounds in a year.

Easy Swap # 7: Have a piece of fruit instead of a candy bar.
You can have this 5 days a week - Lose 10 - 12 pounds in a year.

Healthy Breakfast Ideas

Many of my readers ask about what sort of options I would recommend for a healthy breakfast. I find this can be a problem every day, so I know how hard it can be to find time for a healthy breakfast.

Starting the day with a good breakfast is important. If you begin the day without a meal, then you will find that you have low blood-sugar levels which can impact upon your ability to control cravings. If you let that happen, then you will start wanting a sugar fix, so you'll be tempted to eat a donut or sugary pastry or another unhealthy choice.

The other problem with breakfast is that many typical breakfasts are not as healthy as you need when you want to seriously manage your weight and keep it off for the long term. Here are some of the problems with the selections available for breakfast:

Too much sugar or too many carbs - Breakfast foods such as pancakes, toast, waffles, pastries, donuts, bagels, scones, sugary cereals, pies, breakfast bars or muffins (which in the end are really just cake). The problem with these kind of breakfast options is that they tend to be low in protein and fat, holding nothing but empty carb calories. This then means you are starting the day with a blood-sugar spike, which in turn leads to a quick drop. That sets you up for a roller-coaster of blood-sugar highs and lows all day.

Too much fat - Alternative breakfast options such as fried eggs, bacon, sausages, cheesy omelets, cream cheese on bagels, Egg Mc Muffins, Sausage Mc Muffins, hash browns, any fried English or Scottish style breakfast foods. These types of food simply start the day by giving you a load of fat, which is the fastest way to go over the recommended fat intake through the day.

So what are you left with? Well, there are actually many other options. There are in the following 7 different ideas that will help you to start the day with a healthy and nutritious breakfast. I'm sure that if you look around, you'll find there are many more. Keep an eye out for foods that are low in saturated fats, have whole-grain carbohydrates and also look for low-fat dairy or soy options. When choosing a cereal that will take you through to lunchtime without developing cravings, look for those that have plenty of fiber and essential nutrients.

How do you find the time? The answer is simply to make the time. Try getting up 15 minutes earlier. The quality nutrition you will get from a good breakfast will give you the energy you need to manage the earlier start. If you're really pressed for time, find options that you can pack and have on the way to work. The alternative is to get your breakfast ready the night before. I personally prefer the first option. Starting the day earlier lets you take the time to eat your meal and get the benefits of a slow relaxed meal. As an added bonus, it lets you relax over a nice cup of tea or coffee with your breakfast.

Oatmeal, flaxseed, blueberries & almonds - I think this is an ideal breakfast. Steel-cut oatmeal is the healthiest option, but when you're in a rush, instant oatmeal is fine. The difference is that the instant option has less fiber, but this shouldn't be an issue as the other ingredients have plenty. To prepare this breakfast, microwave the oatmeal and add ground flaxseed, frozen blueberries and sliced almonds. If you like a little extra flavor, some cinnamon and a little honey is a good idea.

This breakfast contains 4 power foods, it's full of fiber, nutrients, protein and good fats. Within just a few minutes preparation, you'll have a healthy, tasty start to the day!

Scrambled tofu - This is a good alternative to scrambled eggs. To give it a bit of extra flavor, you can add onions, peppers or some other veggies. For extra zing - add a little light soy sauce, black powder and garlic powder. Stir-fry the tofu with olive oil and enjoy on some whole-grain toast for a quick, delicious start to the day.

Grapefruit with whole-wheat toast and almond butter - Fresh grapefruit provides you with a great morning 'pick-me-up'. If you find the taste a bit sour, sprinkle a little sugar on top. The almond butter on the toast is healthier than using peanut butter, while the whole grain toast will keep your energy and blood sugar level stable.

Fresh fruit salad - Slice a mixture of apples, berries, pears, oranges, bananas and grapes. Choose whatever you like and add some lemon or lime for a refreshing morning meal. Perfect.

Protein shake with extras - Using your Almased protein powder (or other protein powder) blend low-fat milk or soy milk with some frozen blueberries. You can also add some almond butter or oatmeal as well.

This may sound a little strange, but it is very filling and tasty too! If you haven't any oatmeal, then ground flax seed can work well too.

Eggs with peppers - I don't personally like eggs all that much, but plenty of people enjoy them. If you are trying to keep weight off, then why not try using egg whites instead of the whole egg. These are healthier and you can add some olive oil, green and red bell peppers, broccoli, onions and a little black pepper to taste. The eggs are a good breakfast with some whole-wheat toast.

Cottage cheese and fruit - Low-fat cottage cheese with some added fruit such as apple, citrus or berries is a flavorsome breakfast option with which to start the day.

Sweet facts - What you must know about sugar and carbohydrates

Sugar is one thing that tends to get a bit of a bad rap. Much like fat, sugar gets the blame for a lot of problems - and not everything we're told is 100% correct. Sugars are one type of carbohydrates (carbs), this much is correct. A lot of confusion comes in because people believe carbs are bad. In fact, eating the right kind of carbohydrates is good for you, but the trick is that you need to keep track and make sure you eat them in the right amounts. If we didn't eat carbohydrates, then we would have no energy to get through our day.

In order to succeed at losing weight and keeping it off long term, you should take your time to understand how carbohydrates work and what eating sugar and other carbs means for your energy levels and weight.

The bad reputation that carbohydrates have generally comes from those found in highly processed sugars and starch. At the opposite end of the scale, in fact, there are carbs in broccoli - and no one would argue that this is bad for you! So what you need to know is how you can select the foods that contain the 'good' carbs. Once you know how to tell the difference, you'll be able to enjoy sweet foods, while still maintaining good health and a desirable body weight.

The key to choosing 'good' carbohydrates is to know that they can be found in a wide range of food and there are many different types of sugar. What we put in our coffee or on our cereal is just one type.

Sugars - The good and the bad

Actually, from a nutritional standpoint, there isn't really a 'bad' sugar. Any sugar can be digested and provides the body with energy.

At a cellular level, it makes little difference how glucose gets into your system.

When you take in different types of carbohydrates, they behave differently in the body. The more complex carbohydrates are the better kind for a slow, sustained energy release. These give the body energy over a period of time and provide other nutrition to the body. The 'bad' carbs are the simple kind (such as in processed sugar).

These carbohydrates release energy quickly, increasing your insulin levels (the 'fat' hormone) and leaving you hungry again shortly after taking in the first lot of food. The second type of carbohydrates is typical of what is found in junk food.

'Good' carbs

To ensure that you don't have problems with your weight and to help you to maintain stability within your body and your blood sugar levels - you may opt to eat complex carbohydrates or 'good' carbs. These are the long chains of carbohydrates that your body has to work hard to break down into energy giving glucose. These basic units of energy enter the bloodstream slowly and steadily, which means a stable blood sugar level and a steady flow of energy. That in turn ensures you feel full for longer and you don't experience cravings that can arise when you have sharp highs and lows in sugar levels.

The best complex carbohydrate foods

- Legumes such as peas, beans, lentils and chick peas
- Vegetables such as cabbage and broccoli
- Root vegetables
- Plain oatmeal (with no added sugar)
- Whole grain Pasta
- Soy
- Sweet potatoes or yams
- Whole grains such as brown rice, barley or whole wheat
- Whole-grain cereals

The most satisfying carbohydrates

The list of carbs above not only provide you with energy, these foods will also provide a range of vitamins, minerals and also fiber. You could say you're getting more nutritional 'bang for your buck' when you eat these complex carbohydrates.

When you start each meal with these types of complex carbohydrate foods, then you'll find that you experience considerably less cravings for fatty, sugary food throughout the rest of the meal.

These foods will help you to feel more satisfied, which is exactly the effect of the cabbage soup - and the reason why the diet prepares you to manage your weight for the long term.

The next best carbohydrates

The next step down from complex carbohydrates are the simpler, monosaccharide fructose sugars. While these carbs on their own are absorbed much more rapidly, the 'package' that they come in - fruit - provides fiber which stabilizes their release into the blood stream. Added to that, fruit is a source of vitamins and minerals - so it is a nutritious choice for the body as well.

Fructose differs from simple glucose, because it is diverted to the liver before being released into your system. Fructose is also a good choice of food just before or after exercise, as it contains glycogens (a type of sugar stored in the liver).

'Bad' carbs

One thing to understand is that fructose is in fact quite similar to the sucrose in the white table sugar you add to coffee. What makes it different is that fruits are packaged with vitamins, minerals and fiber. The result is that the fructose reacts differently to sucrose when eaten.

By eating the sugar in fruit, you are having it as nature intended. The extra nutrients and the fiber mean that it is absorbed steadily and the troughs and peaks that can cause havoc with your system are not a problem when you eat sugar that is found in fruit. All these healthy extras are what is removed when you take the type of sugar you find in fruit and process it down to get the kind of sugar found in junk food. It is last refined sugar product that the 'bad' carbohydrates come from.

What are Sugar Blues?

No, it's not some new band! The sugar blues is a physical and emotional state that can occur when you have been eating a lot of refined sugar in highly processed foods. So that you can understand what this is - let's look at the way in which these sugars are processed as they travel through you system.

Simple sucrose molecules in refined sugar are sometimes called 'junk sugars'. They are given this name because these simple carbohydrates are small, uncomplicated molecules that require little effort for processing.

When these molecules are processed in the intestine, there is a rapid release of glucose into the bloodstream. The blood sugar levels rise rapidly and a spike in sugar levels occurs almost immediately.

When this sharp rise in blood sugar occurs, the body immediately tries to compensate by producing and releasing insulin from the pancreas. Insulin is a necessary hormone as it facilitates the uptake of glucose from the blood. However, eating processed sugar, unlike complex carbs and fructose, means a subsequent rapid drop in blood sugar levels. With lots of insulin still buzzing through your system, you then begin to experience hypoglycemia or 'the sugar blues'.

This is when the rollercoaster ride can really start to begin. Now that your body finds that you don't have sufficient blood sugar, the insulin production stops and a range of stress hormones designed to increase blood sugar levels kick in.

The second cycle of hormones sends glucose from the liver back into the blood stream to try to correct the imbalance. Unfortunately, some people find their body can over do things, causing another blood sugar spike - and so the cycle continues... For a number of people, these ups and downs can impact upon their mood - hence the term - sugar blues.

Sweet nothings vs. sweet somethings

There are many different types of sugars. Some sugars are 'sweet somethings', others are 'sweet nothings'. This later group falls into the same category as fake fats. Not only do they deliver no essential nutrients to your body - you would actually be better off without them and they may be doing you harm.
Common sources of 'sweet nothings':

Soft drinks - Soft drinks are actually a double dose of 'nasties'. They combine sugar with caffeine, which can create internal havoc for your body. The biochemical properties of this drink are completely at odds with what your body needs. The caffeine in the soft drink has a diuretic effect. It doesn't relieve your thirst - it increases it! Added to that, a regular can of cola (355 ml or 12.5 oz), holds roughly 10 teaspoons of sugar. If you're taking in a mix like that several times a day - then I'm sure you can see what a recipe for disaster that is.

Another important fact to consider is that when you mix processed sugar into water, the body takes up a higher number of calories and produces more body fat than if you had simply eaten a plain spoonful of dry sugar. The rapid insulin increase that follows causes the liver to turn excess sugar into fats.

Adding caffeine to this mix simply serves to increase the up and down effect and will further stimulate hormones in the body.

Packaged baked goods - Baked goods contain mostly white sugar, white flour and hydrogenated shortening.

This is essentially an 'empty' nutritional package. The problem with packaged bakery goods is that sweet snacks such as cupcakes and donuts, are primarily made from these nutritionally poor ingredients.

The Solution: When you are shopping, look out for baked goods that contain healthy alternatives. This includes whole grains, non-hydrogenated oils and fruit concentrates for sweetness.

Understanding Glycemic Load vs. Glycemic Index

One of the most important things to know when you are evaluating good and bad carbs is their glycemic index. I discussed this briefly in chapter two, but now I'd like to cover it in more detail, as this is very important to understand.

Some important points to consider:

- Eating high GI foods can cause insulin surges, which make people likely to eat 60 - 70% more calories at their next meal.
- When you consume foods that are relatively high in glucose (e.g. white bread, most commercial whole wheat bread or raisins) - you're likely to eat around 200 more calories at your next meal than you would if you'd eaten a meal containing fructose (the sugar in fruit).
- Eating high GI foods leads to elevated insulin and blood glucose levels. This in turn stimulates fat-storage, exacerbates hyperactivity and is likely to reduce sports performance.

GI levels are important when eating carbohydrate rich snacks

When you eat a meal with a variety of carbohydrates types, then GI levels are less important, as eating a variety of different foods means they balance each other out.

When you are having a snack on the other hand, GI becomes much more important. If you ate an apple for example, it would be considered better than a banana as a snack. The lower GI of the apple makes it more blood sugar 'friendly'. A higher GI food like the banana however, would be fine as part of a meal where it's offset by the other foods (e.g. for breakfast).

This is why I suggest you mix the banana with low-fat milk on the banana diet day. Eating the banana with lower GI foods will balance the sugar levels.

Fat and fiber are 2 of the things that slow the absorption of sugar, This means that if you ate an ice cream which contains fat, it would create less of a blood-sugar high than a soda. Likewise, the sugars in a baked potato eaten without sour cream will reach the bloodstream faster than a potato with lashings of butter or sour cream. If you ate a whole orange (which contains fiber), the sugar will enter the bloodstream more slowly than if you had a glass of orange juice and so on. The higher level of fiber also explains why the GI of apples is lower than bananas.

The drinking of soft drinks with a meal works on this same principle; hence the impact of soft drinks on your blood sugar will be less if drunk with a meal rather than drunk on their own.

Bottom Line: GI is a good guideline when selecting foods, however it is important to remember that most of us eat a variety of foods in a meal, not just one food at a time. The main limitation of GI on its own is that it doesn't take into account how the body handles sugar when you eat a variety of foods or have different serving sizes. I recommend that you use glycemic load (GL) as a measure that will provide you with a clearer picture of how food impacts your body and blood sugar levels. If you go back to chapter 2, you can refresh your memory on this - but here is the formula again:

Glycemic Load = Grams of Carbohydrate x GI

By assessing food based upon GL - you get a better idea of the 'real' sugar levels. The consideration of the number of grams of carbohydrate is one way of taking into account the serving size.

Tip: Eating Sweets on a Full Stomach

I've talked about how a 12 oz can of soda can have a more marked impact on insulin levels when taken on an empty stomach. To avoid the insulin spike and adrenalin rush that follows a sugary drink, try drinking the soda with a meal instead. If you like to have a few sweets, then keep the quantities down and have these as a treat after you've eaten a meal to balance the sugar with the other foods. Breakfast choices that are high in sugar are another no-no. Having a breakfast that's high in processed sugar will only set you up for a mid-morning 'crash'.

GI and GL may seem like something that is only important for nutritionists or food scientists, but in the end it is about your health and wellbeing.

If you want to apply this, remember to take note of how your body reacts and use this as your guide. You know best how you feel and behave after eating high GI or GL foods, so you should be best at determining what will work for you.

Tip: Three "Sweet" Beans

If you know that you feel uncomfortable following a sugary meal, then this is likely to be a sign that you're a little sugar-sensitive. I recommend having some three-bean salad. The combination of kidney beans, chickpeas and pinto beans delivers nutrition and proteins in low GI foods. That means no rush of sugar - just steady, stable nutrition.

All About Artificial Sweeteners

The use of artificial sweeteners such as saccharine and aspartame originally came about so that diabetics could have something sweet without creating health issues. It didn't take long before the manufacturers realized that these products had a huge market with dieters.

With so many people believing sugar was so unhealthy, the manufacturers had an eager number of buyers.

I've previously mentioned that artificial sweeteners are no substitute for sweets or carbohydrates. One downside to these sweeteners is that as you become used to them, you can end up wanting more sweet things not less. Your taste buds get used to the flavor and want more and more to satisfy that taste for sugar. By restoring a balance between sweet and savory foods, you'll regain your ability to truly taste the sweetness, so you need less of it to feel satisfied.

Some scientists have expressed worries about the biochemical behaviors of various artificial sweeteners. One worrying examples is aspartame (Nutrasweet). This holds a combination of 2 amino acids which act upon the brain in an altered way to sugars. Although naturally occurring, these amino acids usually enter the brain alongside other nutrients. When they enter alone (as they do in aspartame), this has an unnatural effect on the cells, in particular the neurotransmitters.

A further problem with artificial sweeteners, is that people drink a high number of the drinks they are used in. Earlier I told you about how regular soda will go some way to satisfying the appetite. The problem with artificially sweetened beverages is that they don't 'deliver on their promise'.

They fool your body into thinking that sugar is on the way, then it never arrives. Add to that the fact that they introduce confusing amino acids in a way that wouldn't naturally happen - and you are facing a situation that common sense tells us is not good. Let's face it, introducing unnatural substances to the brain can't be good - whichever way you look at it!

What we really need is to lose our sweet tooth. Instead of trying to create something better than what nature has provided - learn to love the healthy options that are available and you'll soon see the benefits. If you cut out the processed sugar, you'll find you need less of a good thing to be satisfied (that's less calories, by the way!), PLUS you'll enjoy a little a lot more. You could be sitting down to a bowl of naturally sweet and juicy raspberries, drizzled with melted dark chocolate and enjoying something really decadent and healthy… We all just need to learn to say no to every donut that comes our way!

Aspartame and artificial sweeteners are not the solution - my recommendation if you are having doubts is to leave it.

Healthy ways to satisfy your sweet tooth

If you have a sweet tooth and you often reach for the sugar bowl to add a little sugariness to dishes, then I've got put together these hints to help you satisfy your sweet tooth the healthy way!

Cinnamon - With this sweet spice you'll find a little goes a long way.

Just 2 teaspoons will sweeten a tart apple pie, cutting the amount of sugar you'll need to add. Unlike sugar that has 'empty' calories, cinnamon also contains traces of vitamin B, fiber, iron and calcium!

Other sweet spices - Using various spices to add some real flavor to your cooking will cut out the need to add sugar every time. Great options to use include cloves, anise, ginger and mint. A slice of lemon or a twist of lemon peel can really 'lift' a range of beverages, even plain filtered water.

Fruit toppings - I've mentioned the fact that fruit contains fructose, which is similar to the sugar in your sugar bowl. If you want something sweet without the empty calories or a sky high GI - then try crushed pineapple, apple sauce, strawberries or blueberries on your pancakes or waffles. To really bring out the full flavor of the fruit, sprinkle it with some nutmeg or cinnamon.

Plain yogurt flavored with fresh fruits - this is a great alternative to fruit preserves and has a natural, healthy sweetness.

Unsweetened frozen fruit - This is a much better alternative to canned or preserved fruit which may have a lot of added sugar.

Reduce the sugar in your recipes by half - If the recipe requires a lot of sugar, look for a reduced sugar version or add cinnamon, nutmeg, vanilla or fruit concentrate to give it added sweetness. Recipes that require a lot of sugar can often be altered to reduce this - for example, if a recipe needs 1 cup of sugar, try using 1/4 cup to 1/2 cup of honey.

Tip: Try replacing your sugar in a tea or coffee with a cinnamon stick. Stirring your drink keeps your hands occupied and helps you to cut down on sugar.

A cinnamon stick can also be a good way to help you kick the after meal sugar habit and even help you to quit smoking!

Get The Real Facts About Food & Detect Food Manipulation

Learning to understand good health and the role of nutrition will free you to achieve the weight you desire and maintain it. The diet week is the first step on the path to success, so now I'd like to help you understand more about how to follow on after that week. One of the most important things you must learn is how the food industry and media, as well as political, cultural and social influences play a part in food manipulation.

How today's food is different

We've all heard the catch-cry - "does this make me look fat?" or "I'm watching my weight" - but there it is a very real concern for many people. Today 2 in every 3 people in the US is now overweight. It almost seems impossible to think that 2/3 of the population can fall into this category, but it's true.

So the question is - what's causing this to happen? Well here's a big hint… The Center for Disease Control and Prevention has identified that the American male eats some 7% more calories each day than in 1971. The story is even worse for women. American females on average eat a whopping 18% more calories. That's an extra 335 calories a day. In real terms, that's enough to gain 1 pound every 11 days! So the question is - how did this happen?

No, our stomachs haven't expanded - none of us have changed, but our food has.

Our traditional foods are much higher in calories

Early on the 70s, food manufacturers came across a cheap replacement for sugar. What they introduced was a high-fructose corn syrup (HFCS). Today this HCFS is found in a broad range of different foods – it is present in foods ranging from breakfast cereals to bread, pasta sauce to ketchup, from fruit juice to ice tea.

The FDA believes that the average American now takes in 82 g (2.9 oz) of added sugar per day. That makes an additional 317 empty calories in our day to day diet. HFCS is not any worse for our bodies than normal sugar, but with its low cost and sweeping introduction into such a wide range of foods, it is little wonder that America's sweet tooth has grown in recent times.

Supersizing our bodies - not just our meal size

Being conscious of our money, especially in tough financial times, we see the words 'value meal' and we take advantage of this. If you have ever been offered an upsize on an order, then think a little more carefully about what that really means. The supersizing of a large number of fast foods means that we can now get an extra 73% in calories for just 17% more money. That might sound like a great deal, but the reality is, we probably don't need that extra 73% in calories.

About Trans Fat

A generation ago, baked goods had a very short 'shelf life', so manufacturers started looking for a way to produce foods that would keep longer. One big problem was that baked foods needed oil and this wouldn't last at room temperature.

Manufacturers in the 60s came across a way to prevent this problem with the discovery of Trans Fat. Trans fat meant that it became cheaper and more effective to prepare crisp potato chips, deep fried foods and sweet treats like Oreo cookies. The downside is that the trans fat has a terrible effect on our bodies. It increases LDL (the bad type of cholesterol) and lowers HDL (the good cholesterol). We are now at a much greater risk of heart disease and obesity. On a list of ingredients, the only clue that this is present is the phrase "partially hydrogenated".

In order to make food more appealing and to 'mask' the reality of the situation, we have been manipulated. This food manipulation has also necessitated some manipulation of our minds. We are being sold this idea so that we will spend more of our money on the foods that contain this trans fat - and as a result, we now have a diet that contains far more calories than we would have in the past.

With food and beverages now more dense in calories, it becomes increasingly difficult to find healthy choices from readily available pre-prepared products. Added to that, these items are sold in restaurants and grocery stores, so hunting down the 'good' options can be truly hard work. To help you overcome this, I've put together a range of invaluable resources so that you're able to make the right choices.

Developing a lasting weight loss concept

To ensure that you can successfully stay on top of your weight and achieve your weight loss goals, I'd like to show you how to build upon what you started during the Cabbage Soup Diet 2.0 week.

Comparing a broad range of concepts for weight loss goes beyond the scope of this book, but I'd like to help you to develop positive strategies to ensure ongoing weight loss and ultimately weight stability once you complete the diet week.

For some people, the diet week and the "soup as a starter" strategy is just what they need to get started on a path to long term health and weight control. It is the perfect way for them to lose and manage their weight for the long term. Other dieters find that they are less able to maintain this and are at risk of redeveloping their past bad habits again. For those people, the important thing is to find a lasting weight loss concept. If that sounds like you, then read on!

Four Steps To Help You Slim Down and Keep The Weight Off

Step 1: Gradual exercise

My recommendation is that you don't try to alter your whole life at once. If you want to maximize your success after the diet week, then begin by taking small steps toward your goals. Start by getting active and make a commitment to stick with this every day for a month, for at least 10 or 15 minutes a day.

Some key points for developing an exercise routine:

- **Pick one type of exercise** - If you already have an interest in running, hiking or something else, then you should get started by taking on a very low key, simple exercise program. If you haven't already got an interest, then try out a treadmill, cycling machine, rowing machine, trampolining or even just walking.

  Mix it up a little to stay interested and try and make sure you get moving every day. The important thing is to stay motivated.

- **Start out slowly** - This is one of the most important points. It's great to be enthusiastic, but if you get too carried away, the aches and pains could be enough to get your backing out early on. Start slowly, then build your way up. I find that it can work best to start at about half of what you think you can do; you can always build up from this.

- **Try to do at least a little every day** - A good way to keep up with this is to jot down how you are going in your diet journal. This will help you see that you are keeping on track and it will help you follow your progress as you aim to increase your workout and do more each day.

- **Select a time to do your exercise each day** - The morning is an ideal time, but ultimately, the most important thing is to ensure you do the workout every day, so make sure you do it at a time that works for you.

- **Strength** - Including strengthening exercises will help to improve your fitness and your health. Adding daily strengthening workouts will boost your success. Keep it simple to begin with.
Good options include doing sit-ups, crunches, lunges and squats. Start slowly and use your own body weight for resistance without added weights when exercising.

- **Make a start** - One of the biggest hurdles of all is simply to get started. If you procrastinate then you will not get the added benefits of this regular exercise. When you feel like you lack motivation, gather the energy to just get out the door. Once you actually make a start, you may be surprised how easy it can be to keep going for the duration you were initially aiming for.

Step 2: Keep swapping more fattening foods for healthy choices

This was one of the recommended strategies in chapter 5. I gave you a number of suggestions for making tasty, natural and low fat breakfasts. Now you need to keep going and find other ways to replace processed, fatty foods throughout the rest of your day. Make these changes slowly and steadily, each change takes you one step closer to a healthier lifestyle and your ideal weight.

Some essential points

I find that a good way to start cutting out fatty foods is to begin with a list. Write the top 10 foods that you enjoy, placing your all time favorite - the one you never thing you'll give up - at number 1. Work down to number 10, making this the one you could most easily give up.

Once you have this list, start from the bottom (no. 10) and work your way up. Replace that food with a low-fat option. If you're not sure what to replace it with, go online and look around for something that will suit you. My list of easy-swap options could also help you to get some inspiration. You could be amazed at the variety of low-fat options out there.

If you don't believe that there is a suitable low-fat alternative, give yourself a month to see how you go living without the food. At the end of the month, give yourself a small treat to acknowledge what you've achieved. You can add it back into your diet at the end of the month, but I'm confident you'll find that you didn't need it as much as you thought!

I believe the more you make these changes, the easier it will become. Eating healthy, nutritious food will simply become second nature - and your body will thank you for it!

Reducing fat can also be done easily when you select suitable options to cook with. Cut back on the use of oils, introduce healthier olive oil and use some alternatives such as steaming your vegetables.

I find that using a wok is a great way to lose weight. This traditional Asian cooking utensil is ideal for tasty, low-fat cooking. Try using a strainer to skim excess fat from soups or stews and a low-fat cooking brigade is a great gift each time you manage to eliminate something from your top 10 greasy food list.

Step 3: Introduce more low Glycemic Load foods into your daily diet

The Cabbage Soup Diet is a low Glycemic diet. It contains mostly foods that hold a low Glycemic Value and a low Glycemic Load. These help to stabilize energy levels and eliminate mood swings. By balancing good nutrition with low Glycemic foods, you can reduce your overall hunger and eliminate the urge to 'cheat'.

The following chart is to help you to slowly phase out the foods that are undesirable from your diet. You don't have to make sweeping changes all in one go, but instead find a good balance and work towards improving your overall eating habits.

Desirable Foods	Moderately Desirable	Less Desirable Foods
Breads: whole grain wheat or rye pita bread, coarse European-style, cracked or sprouted whole wheat	**Breads**: pumpernickel, 100% stone ground whole wheat, 100% whole grain rye crisp cracker	**Breads**: white bread, most commercial whole wheat breads, English muffins, bagel, French bread, baguettes, most commercial matzoh
Cereals: compact noodles, high bran cereals (All-Bran, Fiber One), coarse oatmeal, porridge, coarse whole grain (Kashi), cereal mixed with Psyllium (Fiberwise)	**Cereals**: grape-nut cereal, medium-fine grain oatmeal, (5-minute variety)	**Cereals**: corn flakes, puffed rice, puffed wheat, flaked cereals, instant "quick" or pre-cooked cereals. oatbran, rolled oats. shredded wheat, Muesli, refined cereals
Pasta, Grains and Starchy Vegetables: pasta (all types), bulgur, buckwheat (kasha) couscous, kidney beans dry, (lentils, black-eyed peas, chick-peas kidney beans, lima beans, peas, sweet potato, yam (soybeans lowest), amaranth, most vegetables.	**Pasta, Grains and Starchy Vegetables**: brown Rice, boiled potato, corn navy beans, kidney beans (canned), baked beans. beets, carrots.	**Pasta, Grains and Starchy Vegetables**: instant rice, instant precooked grains, baked potato, micro-waved potato, instant potato, winter squash (acorn, butternut), parsnips.

Milk Products:
skim, 1%, cottage cheese, (lowfat or regular), buttermilk, Low-fat plain yogurt, cottage cheese

Milk Products:
2% milk, cheese, regular plain yogurt, low-fat cheese,

Milk Products:
whole milk, ice milk, ice cream, yogurt sweetened with sugar, low-fat frozen desserts with sugar added, low-fat and regular frozen yogurt with sugar added, tofu ice cream.

Fruit:
most fruit and natural fruit juices, including apple, berries, cantaloupe, grapefruit, honeydew, oranges, pears, grapes, peaches, applesauce, cherries, plums, grapefruits.

Fruit:
banana, kiwi, mango, papaya, pineapple, watermelon, orange juice.

Fruit:
raisins, figues, fruit juices sweetened with sugar.

Meats/Meat Replacement:
shellfish, "white" fish (cod, flounder, trout, tuna in water), chicken, turkey, cornish hen, venison (white meat no skin), egg substitutes (cholesterol free), Tofu, Quorn

Meats/Meat Replacement
higher fat fish, (salmon, herring, lean cuts of beef, pork, veal. low-fat imitation luncheon meat, eggs.

Meats:
most cuts of beef, pork, lamb, hot dogs (including "low-fat' versions) cheese, luncheon meats, peanut butter.

Remember, good health and the introduction of low glycemic food is about balance, not undereating or depriving yourself.

To improve your health and manage your weight, the focus by adoption low glycemic foods should be lowering the quantities of foods you eat which increase insulin and stimulate fat-storage.

The goal is not to cut out all high glycemic foods - and nor would you want to. The goal is to instead understand that this list can help you make positive diet choices. Mixing low Glycemic Index foods with small amounts of high glycemic foods is also unlikely to upset the hunger reducing effects.

One good example is carrots. They have a high Glycemic Index, but carry a low Glycemic Load. I recommend these in small quantities as a great option to boost your energy, even during the diet week, as they will not adversely affect your other low Glycemic Index foods by rapidly increasing insulin levels. Having a pound of carrots in one sitting on the other hand, would not be a good idea and could cause elevated insulin levels. This is also the case with water melons.

People with certain body types will find that a simple change from high glycemic food to low glycemic food is enough to bring about a significant loss of body fat, without altering calorific intake.

Working out which variations of low glycemic food you wish to eat is entirely up to you. The key is to ensure you eat enough calories to meet your body's daily need. To give your health a real boost, make sure you have a variety of vegetables, fruits, grains and other foods daily. The wide range of foods will ensure your body receives all the phytochemicals, vitamins and minerals it needs.

Step 4: Increase exercise slowly. After the first month of doing very short, gentler workouts every day, it's now time to begin increasing your daily exercise and start to intensify the exercise.

Here are some points to remember:

- **Duration**: One of the first things to do is begin to increase the duration of the workouts. Continue with low intensity workouts and begin to increase the amount of time you workout. 5 is usually a good start. Increase this for 2-3 workouts, then add a further 5 minutes and so on. Aim to reach about 40-45 minutes each day. (One hour long workout each week is also good.)

- **Intensity**: When you have successfully built up the duration of your workouts, then begin to increase the intensity.

  Initially, you may need to cut back the duration. To manage this, try to then do intervals at a higher intensity. For example, cut your duration from 40 minutes to 20 minutes. Next increase and decrease the intensity at intervals throughout the workout. For example, complete 3-4 minutes at a faster pace, followed by an easier pace, then pick up a faster pace again and so on. An important step to ensure you don't become injured is to do a warm up and a cool down at the end of the workout.

- **Hard-easy variation**: As you increase the duration and intensity of your workouts, vary them by doing one longer workout of 45 minutes followed by a shorter one of 20-25 minutes the following day.

  If you are doing interval workouts, then do these on one day with a shorter, easier workout the next. The longer, more intense workouts are the 'hard' days, while the shorter, less intensive workouts are the easy days. Always alternate these so that you don't cause yourself injury or overdo things.

Stay on track today, tomorrow, and for the rest of your life

Did you know that when you eat a heavy, fatty meal your body needs more energy to digest this than when you eat plenty of fruit and vegetables. This is why many of us experience feelings of lethargy following a heavy meal. Digestion can steal a lot of energy and this is why plenty of fruit and vegetable is useful. They are easily digested and have many useful nutrients as well.

Eating fruit and vegetables provides you with more energy and a greater sense of well being. When you come through the cabbage soup diet, you'll feel the positive effects of this.

With the techniques that I've covered in chapter 5 and chapter 6, you'll also begin to automatically start changing your diet to a more alkaline one. With all the extra quantities and varieties of fruits, vegetables and salads - you'll be on the right track to a new, effervescent and energetic you.

These things will help you to feel healthier and happier - plus they will
support you slim down. Did you know that the secret to many people's slim,
fit appearance and enhanced vitality is that they eat 5 portions of fruit and vegetables every day?

These days, around 70% of my nutrition is sourced from fruits and vegetables. Before making this change, I could never have imagined what an incredible amount of energy I would get from this.

Our bodies are genetically programmed consume a range of vital nutrients

The nutrition that was available to us in the Stone Age came from a highly diverse range of fresh, 100 % natural produce. Everything we ate was free from contaminants, meat was fat-free and there was definitely no use of hormones in the production. Our diets consisted mostly of fruits, berries, roots, mushrooms and the green parts of plants. This was then supplemented with small game, eggs and fish.

When analyzing what we believe our forebears ate, it indicates that their diet held three times the nutrition level of what we eat today. Linus Paulin, originator of orthomolecular medicine, believes that our ancestors are likely to have consumed up to 30 times more of some vitamins. The point is this - our bodies have adapted and evolved to consume certain nutrient levels over a period of around 4 million years.

Because of this extended period of evolution we adapted us for a particular diet and nutrition level.

Our bodies simply cannot process high levels of fat and sugar which have only been present in our diets a relatively short time, since we have been eating 'industrial' food. These foods are often lacking in vital nutrients - which is how many experts explain the overwhelming desire to overeat.

An alarming number of overweight and obese people are in fact malnourished. They overeat because the foods they chose lack the essential vitamins and minerals they require.

The result is that they gain weight, but their bodies crave more - compelling them to eat in an effort to try to get those essential nutrients. So the question is - how do you know which foods to chose to ensure you have that essential nutrition?

Using the latest, scientific food pyramid

If you are unsure about what you should be eating to get the nutrition you need, then my advice is to follow a food pyramid. These diagrammatical representations emerged as a guideline to help people make choices about food. Earlier pyramids, such as the U.S. government's Food Guide Pyramid and similar ones from that era are unfortunately now out of date as our understanding of nutrition has changed, or they were based upon certain commercial interests.

There is, however, an up to date alternative - and that is the Healthy Eating Pyramid created by the faculty of the Department of Nutrition at the Harvard School of Public Health. This pyramid is based on the latest science, without any business interests having an influence upon its guidelines, plus it was updated in 2008.

I recommend that you follow this pyramid if you wish to understand the latest ideas from recent research into healthy eating. This one is a straightforward, non-biased representation of a healthy diet.

The Harvard developed Healthy Eating Pyramid corrects a number of inherent flaws in the USDA pyramid. It provides more accurate and recent information about how to choose wisely when selecting foods. The basis of this pyramid is a focus on daily exercise and sensible weight control, stressing the connection between these two important elements.

At the base of the pyramid are the foods you should eat most often, vegetables, whole grains etc. and those you should eat the least are at the top, red meat, refined grains, sugary drinks and so on.

A similar approach shows the Danish Food pyramid on the next page.

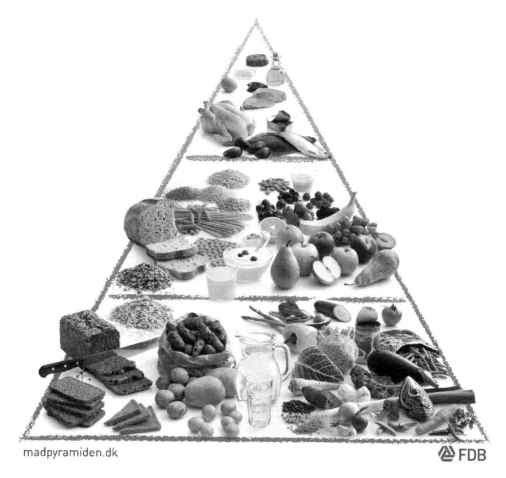

madpyramiden.dk   FDB

Source: Creative Commons, FDB

Following the Healthy Eating Pyramid guidelines - 4 Quick tips

1. Start with exercise. A healthy diet goes hand in hand with regular exercise, keeping calories in balance and your weight in check. I've given you dozens of ideas in this book to help you fit exercise into your life.

2. Focus on food, not grams. The Healthy Eating Pyramid isn't about specific serving sizes or grams of food. It's a simple, straightforward guide to choosing more of the good stuff and cutting back on the bad stuff when you eat.

3. Go with plants. Eating a plant-based diet is the healthiest option. Eat plenty of vegetables, fruits, whole grains and healthy fats, like olive oil. Purchase the best quality oils you can and get adventurous about trying out new delicious, healthy recipes that will bring the Healthy Eating Pyramid into your kitchen and home.

4. Cut way back on American staples. Unfortunately, many of the red meat, refined grains, sugary drinks and salty snacks that are a part of American culture are also very unhealthy. I can't stress enough the need to switch to a plant-based diet - rich in non-starchy vegetables, fruits and whole grains. If you still desire meat, reduce your portions and mix things up with some fish and poultry choices.

The Building Blocks of the Healthy Eating Pyramid

The following are the essential building blocks of the Healthy Eating Pyramid:

Whole Grains

Whole grains are the best source of carbohydrates for energy. Brown rice, oatmeal and whole wheat bread deliver the inner (germ) and outer (bran) layers along with energy-rich starch. These whole grains provide the body with slow release energy, as it can't digest whole grains as quickly as processed carbohydrates such as white flour. That means you feel full for longer and your blood sugar and insulin levels stay stable instead of rising and falling quickly.

Healthy Fats and Oils

Traditionally, we thought that cutting out all fats and oils was essential. However, our bodies require some fats and oils. Healthy oils (generally plant based oils) include olive, corn, soy, peanut, sunflower, and other vegetable oils.

We can also get the necessary healthy oils and fats from non trans fat margarine, butter (1 teaspoon a couple of times a month), nuts, seeds, avocados and fatty fish like salmon.

Vegetables and Fruits

Weight loss is only one benefit of eating a diet filled with plenty of organic fruit and vegetables. Eating these highly nutritious foods can also help to reduce the likelihood of heart attack or stroke, help to protect your body from some types of cancers, lower blood pressure, avoid painful intestinal ailments such as diverticulitis, reduce your risk of bowel cancer and guard against cataract and macular degeneration (the major causes of vision loss among people over age 65). Fruit and vegetables also bring variety to your diet and provide your body with essential fiber.

An added bonus is that natural, organic fruit and vegetables are environmentally more sustainable.

Nuts, Seeds, Beans and Tofu

Nuts, beans, seeds and tofu are all plant based foods as well - and are great sources of protein, fiber, vitamins and minerals. You can use a wide variety of beans, including black beans, navy beans, garbanzos, lentils - and many other beans are also available to use to add interest to your food. Nuts are also a good source of the healthy fats mentioned previously. Try adding a small number of almonds, walnuts, pecans, peanuts, hazelnuts or pistachios to your diet.

Fish, Poultry and Eggs

Another important source of protein is eggs, fish and poultry. There is a mountain of research which demonstrates that eating fish reduces the risk of heart disease and delivers heart-healthy omega-3 fats. Poultry such as chicken and turkey provide essential proteins and are low in saturated fat. Eating eggs used to be considered a bad move - but you could say they're not as bad as they've been cracked up to be! Egg yolk should still be eaten in smaller quantities, but egg whites are very high in protein. If you are at risk of heart disease or diabetes, you should only have the yolks up to 3 times a week, but if you enjoy eggs - then double up the amount of egg white as a substitute to whole eggs in omelets or baking.

Dairy (1 to 2 Servings Per Day) or Vitamin D/Calcium Supplements

Losing weight, building healthy bones and keeping strong requires calcium, vitamin D and exercise. Dairy foods are a great source of nutrients for healthy bones. Eat mostly non-fat or low-fat dairy products for these nutrients. If you don't enjoy dairy products or they don't agree with you, then drinking Almased with water or taking a vitamin D and calcium supplement will help you to ensure you have your daily vitamin D and calcium needs met.

15 more tips to KEEP the NEW YOU permanently!

I've had so many great suggestions from readers on how to keep the weight off for the long term - I'd like to share with you **15 Tried & Tested Tips** from those readers. Each of these weight loss tips has been tried by readers just like you! You may use one, several or all of them depending on what works for your individual situation.

Weight Loss Tip 1: Eat breakfast daily

I provided some great ideas for having a healthy breakfast - but this is also one of the most common pieces of advice from other readers. If you find it hard to find the time for breakfast, then remember that you can at least have a Protein Shake to kick-start the day and keep hunger at bay for 4 hours.

Weight Loss Tip 2: Have a small snack every 3 - 4 hours

A small healthy snack every 3 - 4 hours will keep your metabolism performing at the optimal level. The snack could be apples, oranges, baked pretzels, a handful of seeds and nuts and so on. The choice is yours, but small quantities of healthy food will help to ensure you don't get hungry and develop the urge to overeat.

Weight Loss Tip 3: Try eating two pieces of fruit or vegetable before every meal

If you want to have more variety or you don't always feel like soup or a salad before your meal, then exchange that for two pieces of fruit or vegetable. These are ideal to fill your stomach in a similar way to the soup, helping you to cut down the calories.

Weight Loss Tip 4: Eat at regular intervals

The best idea of all is to have a schedule and stick to it. Eating irregular times can throw things out of balance and upset your whole diet. With a schedule, you can stick to your plan and stay on track to lose weight and keep it off.

Weight Loss Tip 5: NEVER skip your meals. NEVER!

When you skip a meal, you might fool yourself that you're cutting out calories. Unfortunately, it doesn't work that way. When you skip meals, your body starts to slow your metabolism and prepares to store as much energy (fat) as possible at the next meal. What happens is not that you cut calories, but that you cause your body to hold on to as much of what you digest as possible, which ultimately will lead to weight gain rather than weight loss. If you are skipping meals due to time pressures, then try having a protein shake instead.

Weight Loss Tip 6: Eat slowly and thoroughly chew every bite

I recommended this during the diet week, but many readers stress not to forget this after you complete that week. Chewing slowly and savoring your food helps you to eat less and enjoy it more.

Focus on what you are doing, keep your mind on the experience of eating while you are chewing your food. Enjoy the feeling of eating food and allow your body to let you know as you become full. This focus and the feelings you can enjoy as you eat will help to intensify the flavor and you will find that eating becomes almost a ritual, instead of something to be done in a rush.

Weight Loss Tip 7: Keep selecting foods that are fresh, not processed

This is a really useful tip, because in the end, fresh foods not only provide you with higher levels of nutrition, they are also less fattening. Here are some good examples of the kinds of choices you need to make: Potatoes versus chips, Whole Wheat Bread versus Donuts etc. If you're still looking for inspiration, then take another look at my list of overseen goldmines.

Weight Loss Tip 8: Buy pre-cut fruits and vegetables

The thing about fast foods and pre-packaged options is that they're convenient. Many readers have recommended buying pre-cut fruit and vegetables, so that they can compete for convenience.

If you're feeling lazy or you just want something in a hurry, then having a pre-cut option will help you to put together a salad or snack quickly and easily.

Weight Loss Tip 9: Sweeten your food with spice

I've recommended this option - and so do lots of readers just like you! Spices like cinnamon and vanilla are a great way to put a little extra sweetness into your desserts without adding more sugar - plus they're less fattening.

Weight Loss Tip 10: Limit alcohol intake

Start reducing alcohol as it is very fattening and it can quickly reduce your will power to stick to healthy eating. Have alcohol only on special occasions and you will be helping your body not only by reducing your weight, but by avoiding a number of the other side effects of drinking.

Weight Loss Tip 11: Target the "easy wins"

If you were to eat a turkey sandwich with lettuce, tomato and mustard in place of a roast beef sandwich with mayonnaise just twice a week - it could equate to 15 pounds of weight loss in a year!

Weight Loss Tip 12: Make the most of beans

Beans are a great source of proteins and a number of other nutrients. Finding ways to include these in your diet will help to boost your overall health and nutrient levels. An example would be to add a handful beans to your salads or soups to help you feel fuller and curb your hunger pangs for longer.

Weight Loss Tip 13: Drink either before or after your meal

It is important to drink plenty either before or after you eat. If you drink while you're eating, it can cause you to overeat and not recognize when you are full. The best option is to drink plenty either before you start or when you are finished.

Weight Loss Tip 14: Supplement it

Many readers find that a herbal supplement helps to boost their diet success and curb their appetite. A good herbal supplement or vitamin supplement can also boost your energy, helping to limit any urge to overeat. Almased is a great supplement as it does all these things.

Weight Loss Tip 15: The last and final tip - FOLLOW ALL THE ABOVE TIPS!

Losing weight can be best achieved when you learn to listen to your body and pick up on those signs or indicators about what you need to eat and when. There are few absolute musts in the Cabbage Soup Diet, because I want it to be easy and in particular, I want it to help you start preparing yourself to make good decisions in the future.

Using these tips above is part of that process of adopting a positive view to long term health, then building on losing weight from there.

Some final words

The Cabbage Soup Diet 2.0 is perfect for putting you on the fast track to quick weight loss. After you complete the diet week and start shedding those pounds and inches, I want to see you start making positive changes and implementing long term strategies from the tips you have here. With those strategies in place, you'll be on the right path to creating your own custom made, long-term weight loss plan - a plan that will truly be about what works for you!

Simplifying things and selecting fresh, tasty food is much easier than you may imagine - like so many things - it is just a case of getting started! Once you take that first step and begin to see the outstanding results, staying on track and motivated couldn't be easier.

The Healthy Eating Pyramid really is an incredible tool and one that will help you to achieve far better results. The guidelines in this pyramid are an indicator of optimal nutrition levels - giving you energy to exercise and stay mentally focused on your goal. Long term weight loss and maintenance is the key - it means not only an improved appearance, but better health inside and out. Following the Cabbage Soup Diet 2.0 and then building upon this starting point with the many hints, tips, techniques, ideas and strategies in this ebook will make you fitter, healthier, slimmer and happier - now and in the future.

One last thought

My vision is to create a resource for dieters who've completed this guide. I hope to build a specific cabbage soup diet 2.0 website that will offer the ideas, help and support of people just like you. By forming a virtual support community, I aim to provide all Cabbage Soup Dieters with a chance to share with others and help them as they start down the road to weight loss and improved health (anonymously if you wish).

If you'd like to be a part of this, then please send your experience. Fill in my contact form on my website:

www.successful-diet-cabbage-soup.com/contact-form.html .

I wish you all the best with your diet efforts and hope you will greatly benefit from the information you have allowed me to share with you. I look forward to hearing how you do.

More options to stay in touch with me

 www.facebook.com/cabbagesoupdiet

 www.youtube.com/user/cabbagesoupdiet20

 www.twitter.com/cabbagesoupdiet

 www.pinterest.com/cabbagesoupdiet/

 www.successful-diet-cabbage-soup.com/Diet-Cabbage-Soup.xml

References and recommended reading:

The successful cabbage soup diet
www.successful-diet-cabbage-soup.com

The New Cabbage Soup Diet,
Margit Danbrot, St. Martin's Paperbacks, (1997)

The Big Healthy Soup Diet,
Linda Lazarides, Harper Thorsons (2005)

The Volumetrics Weight-Control Plan
Barbara J. Rolls and Robert A. Barnett, Mass Market Paperback,
(Dec 31, 2002)

Die magische Kohlsuppe
Marion Grillparzer, Gräfe & Unzer; (March, 2006)

Eat this not that
David Zinczenko and Mat Goulding, Rodale Books; Upd Exp edition
(October 6, 2009)

Eat, Drink, and Be Healthy:
The Harvard Medical School Guide to Healthy Eating Simon &
Schuster,
June 2001, by Harvard School of Public Health professor and
researcher Walter Willett, M.D.

Are Toxins fattening?
Elisabeth Hsu-LeBlanc
www.dinakhader.metacanvas.com

Food Pyramids – What should you really eat?
www.hsph.harvard.edu/nutritionsource/what-should-you-eat/
pyramid-full-story/index.html

Kindle Editions by Gabriela Rupp

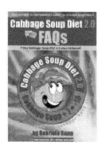
Cabbage Soup Diet 2.0 - FAQs
[Kindle Edition]
Gabriela Rupp

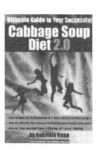
Cabbage Soup Diet 2.0 –
The Ultimate Guide
[Kindle Edition]
Gabriela Rupp

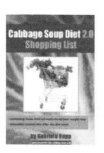
Cabbage Soup Diet 2.0 -
Shopping List
[Kindle Edition]
Gabriela Rupp

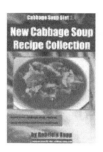
Cabbage Soup Recipes 2.0
[Kindle Edition]
Gabriela Rupp

Made in United States
Orlando, FL
09 July 2022

19576535R00076